THE STRANGE MEDICAL SAGA OF JOHN F. KENNEDY

By

Forest Tennant

Published by the
Tennant Foundation
West Covina,
California

ISBN: 9781955934213
Library of Congress Control Number: 2023903440

Special discounts are available on quantity purchases by corporations, associations, educators, and others. For details, contact one of the parties listed below.

U.S. trade bookstores and wholesalers: Please contact
Nancy Kriskovich Tel: (406)249-2002;
or email snkriskovich@gmail.com

All proceeds from the sale of this book will go to the Medical Study and Education Projects sponsored by the
Tennant Foundation
336-338 S. Glendora Ave.
West Covina, CA 91790-3043
Ph: 626-716-2689
Fax: 626-919-7497
Email: tennantfoundation92@gmail.com

ACKNOWLEDGEMENTS

This book could not have been researched and written without the technical assistance of Becky and Tom Marino and Nancy Kriskovich.

DEDICATION

This book is dedicated to the US Military Officers who have served their country in a medical crisis as exemplified by Dr. (Admiral) George G. Burkley who cared for three President, Eisenhower, Kennedy and Johnson.

ABOUT THE COVER

The cover picture is John F. Kennedy with Dr. William Meninger who founded the Meninger Mental Health Hospital. JFK had a keen desire to improve the nation's mental health. JFK is in a rocking chair prescribed by his primary physician at the time, Dr. Janet Travell. Rocking chair therapy is recognized as having many therapeutic benefits for persons with painful spine disorders.

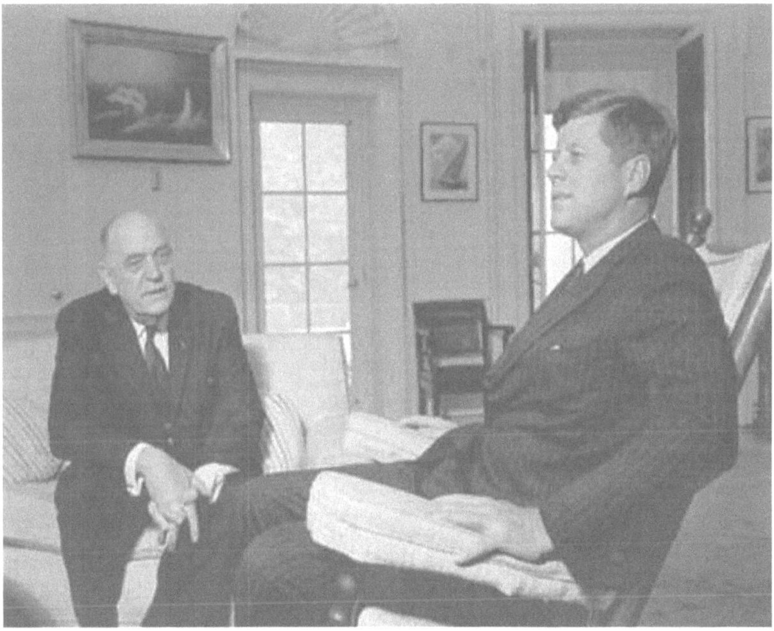

Author's Note

I have chosen to write this book because John F. Kennedy (JFK) has a medical history that can only be called a "strange medical saga." Many excellent components of his medical history have been published. This book pulls these components into a singular, medical history. His medical history is not only a rarity in itself but one of courageous physicians and a strong "will-to-live" on the part of JFK.

JFK was assassinated on November 22, 1963, almost 60 years ago. Since that time some of America's best historians and medical investigators have written parts of JFK's medical saga. Some expert physician investigators have in recent years determined the underlying causes of his medical conditions. Scientific information about these causes wasn't available during JFK's lifetime. This book could not have been written except for some excellent books and investigations. Renowned historian Robert Dallek and his medical consultant, Dr. Jeffrey Kelman in 2002 were the first to review JFK's medical records at the John F. Kennedy Library and Museum. Since then, other researchers have examined JFK's medical records. Of special note and recognition is that Dr. Lee Mandel, a Naval Endocrinologist, was allowed, on three occasions in May and July of 2008, to examine the records. In 2009 Dr. Mandell published his conclusion that JFK was born with autoimmune polyglandular syndrome. This syndrome wasn't named and characterized until the 1980's some 18-20 years after JFK died. Neurosurgeons T. G. Pait and J. T. Dandy have described the methods and results of JFK's back surgeries. Dr. Charles Burton, the renowned neurosurgeon, recognized that JFK developed a rare and extremely painful spine condition called adhesive arachnoiditis. JFK developed this condition due to myelogram dye used to x-ray his spine in the early 1940's.

Historians Richard Lertzman and William J. Birney wrote the bibliography of Dr. Max Jacobson who prescribed performance enhancing drugs to JFK. Susan E. B. Schwartz wrote about the most unknown and unappreciated of JFK's physicians, Dr. Hans Kraus, who was a muscle and strength building genius who literally saved JFK from a terrible downfall in the middle of his presidency. Dr. Janet Travell published her autobiography "Office Hours Day and Night." At the time she started care of JFK in 1955, she was probably the world's greatest pain and rehabilitation specialist. Robert Kennedy said JFK would never have been President if it weren't for Dr. Travell. After JFK's assassination Dr. George Lundberg, a former military pathologist and editor of the Journal of the American Medical Association, along with his partner Dennis Breo interviewed and published the findings of the two pathologists who did JFK's autopsy. They concluded that JFK was killed by two bullets from the rear. They found that JFK had essentially absent adrenal glands which confirmed the long-held belief that he had Addison's Disease.

This book describes JFK's strange medical saga from birth to death. It is a one-of-a-kind, strange medical saga. It compels a new look at JFK and the history he carried.

Prologue

Ask anyone in the public about John F. Kennedy's health and you will get a vague answer about "Addison's Disease," hurt his back in PT109, or "they lied about who and what killed him." The sadness, disdain, and conspiracies that surround JFK's life and assassination have obscured his strange medical saga. He was born with a rare genetic disease and acquired another one. Partly out of fear and partly due to the mysterious, unknown nature of his diseases, his family, political handlers, and physicians felt secrecy about his health conditions was warranted. They particularly didn't want the public to know he had been given "last rites" two times before he became President. Naturally, everyone wants to know what happened and why. Some 50 to 60 years after his death, medical science, in its usual "thrust forward style" has determined the rare diseases that caused his strange medical saga. You will likely have some new beliefs and thoughts about America in the 20th Century when you read this book.

Table of Contents

1. Introduction

A Surprise Inauguration

January 20, 1961, was no ordinary day in Washington, D.C. Eight inches of thick wet snow had fallen overnight. The US Army had to clear the roads with flamethrowers. Although the sun was shining, a harsh skin-burning wind buffeted a crowd of twenty thousand who braved the weather to observe the Inauguration of John F. Kennedy (JFK), the thirty fifth, and, at the age of forty-three, the second youngest to be President of the United States.

To bear the weather, spectators wrapped themselves in whatever they could to stay warm – blankets, sweaters, winter coats, and even sleeping bags. But not JFK. He seemingly ignored the cold and removed his overcoat prior to speaking. He stood over six feet tall, and without coat, hat, scarf, or gloves he exuded the picture of good health and vigor. The fact was that this image was an act and ploy to hide his extremely poor health and sickness. He had already been administered the last rites of the Catholic church on two occasions. About eighty million people were watching the inaugural on television and they needed to know they had elected a fit and healthy President. Unknown to the public, his two personal physicians were in the crowd of spectators. He was deeply indebted and grateful to both. One had clearly saved his life and the other given him enough strength and vitality to wage his Presidential campaign and stand in the cold and give his inaugural speech.

In January 1961, JFK was far too ill to let his key physicians be too far away. Both of his personal physicians at his inauguration were remarkable medical innovators who had brought JFK to this point in his life by the use of little known and non-standard medical treatments. Little known to the public and even to most medical professionals are some of his physicians' innovations. Some have been adopted in modern medicine, and others have been highly criticized and condemned.

JFK was assassinated at the age of forty-six on November 20, 1963. During his life, his family, physicians, and close confidants guarded his health issues in great secrecy. The glamour, charisma, and popularity of he and his wife, Jackie, and the conspiracy theories that continue to surround his assassination have essentially buried his strange medical saga. The average citizen may have heard he had Addison's Disease, and survived PT-109, but that's about it. In actuality, he was born with a rare genetic disease which produced complications that were aggravated by his lust for excitement, competitiveness, and leadership. Being born into extreme wealth and affluence, he and his family were able to seek out the best and most innovative physicians of the day. He was a sickly child and suffered a multitude of medical issues during his life. By fate, with a number of strange quirks, his health in the year he died was probably the best in his adult life.

2. The Beginning: May 29, 1917

Born With Genetic Defects

The beginning of his strange medical saga was on May 29, 1917, when he was born into Boston wealth and high society. No one knew when he passed through his mother's birth canal, that he carried a rare genetic disease. In 1917, physicians had never heard of "autoimmune polyglandular syndrome" which he had but wasn't known until long after his death in 1963. His birth took place in an upstairs bedroom of the Kennedy family home in the Boston suburb of Brookline, Massachusetts. He was the second of nine children born to Rose and Joe Kennedy between 1915 and 1932. Joseph Patrick Kennedy and Rose Elizabeth Fitzgerald, married in 1914 to form a perfect union of Boston's elite Irish class. Twenty-four-year-old Rose, who had been a Boston debutante, and twenty-six-year-old Joe, who had graduated from Harvard and established himself as the city's youngest bank President, looked forward to privileged lives as upper-middle-class Bostonians. Joe's ambitions, however, reached beyond his local moorings to project him onto the national scene. Speculation in stocks after World War I made Joe a millionaire and opened the way to his accumulation of additional millions in the movie industry and the liquor business after the end of Prohibition in 1933.

JFK was also born into a family of talented and astute politicians. His grandfather, John E. Fitzgerald, was elected to the Massachusetts State Senate, three terms as a US Congressman and repeated service as Boston's mayor. His nickname was Fitzie, or "Honey Fitz" and he was known for his captivating personality and gift of gab. Traits that his grandson, JFK, would inherit.

His father, Joe, was also a natural politician. He was not only one of America's wealthiest businessmen, he made substantial financial contributions to the Democratic Party and Franklin Roosevelt's Presidential election campaign. Consequently, Joe was appointed as the first chairman of the Securities and Exchange Commission in 1934, and in 1937 was appointed chair of the U.S. Maritime Commission. Later that year he became ambassador to Great Britain. Although Joe's close identification with Neville Chamberlain's failed appeasement policies in regard to Germany would bring an end to his personal political ambitions, his term as ambassador to Great Britain won his family a place in the Social Register, and this achievement gave him lifelong satisfaction.

There was evidence at birth that JFK inherited significant disease states. One leg was shorter than the other. This asymmetry predisposed him to back pain in adulthood. Later in his life he required a three-eighths inch heal lift in his left shoe to offset the difference in his leg lengths. Later it was known that his back had genetic defects. Joan and Clay Blair wrote a classic book and detailed history in 1976 called "The Search for JFK." They were able to discern that JFK received much of his medical care at the Lahey Clinic in Boston. This clinic, founded in 1925, was considered very prestigious and recruited excellent physicians. Consequently, the rich and famous flocked to the clinic including the Kennedy family. The Blair's learned that Dr. Elmer Bartels had treated JFK for several reasons when he was employed at the Lahey Clinic. Although retired, Dr. Bartels gave the Blair's some critical information relative to the medical saga of JFK. He told them that JFK was "born with an unstable back."

Dr. Bartels went on to explain. "An unstable back is something you are born with, and it doesn't maintain itself properly." An unstable back lasts a lifetime. It is a back that can be normal for long periods of time and then go out of whack for no apparent reason. When it goes out of whack, the pain can be excruciating, lasting days or weeks. During the 1920's and 1930's there was not much anybody could do about an unstable back. The standard treatment was: take it easy. Don't do anything rough or violent to aggravate the back. Take hot baths. In some cases, doctors recommended a type of stiff back brace resembling a corset. Very few recommended surgeries as surgery was considered a "radical" approach. It was not often successful.

Although the term "unstable back" is not an official medical term or diagnosis and hardy recognized today, most every practicing doctor has a general understanding of what it means. It has sometimes been defined as a "congenital malformation of the spinal column with an attendant lifetime disability." There may be some structural, anatomic abnormality that overstretches, slips, or entraps some nerves causing great pain and impairment, but no specific defect has ever been assigned to "unstable back." In fact, however, there are no magnetic resonance imaging (MRI) or myelograms studies that have specifically determined which anatomical part may "wear out." There are probably multiple anatomic defects that can give you an "unstable back" including some that can, as in the case of JFK, worsen with injury or disease with the passage of time. At some point in his teenage or college years, JFK started to periodically wear a back brace or corset which would continue through the rest of his life.

Being born into a wealthy, large prominent family was most fortuitous. On May 29, 1917, no one knew the hazardous and precarious medical conditions that would soon befall JFK and plague him throughout the 46 years of his life. Fortunately, his wealth and intellect allowed him to have the nutrition, education, and medical care that he later required to survive his obvious and not-so-obvious genetic conditions.

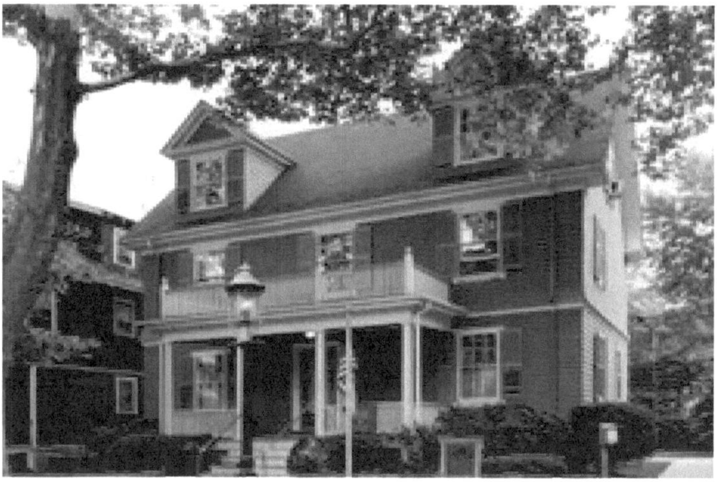

Kennedy's birthplace in Brookline, Massachusetts

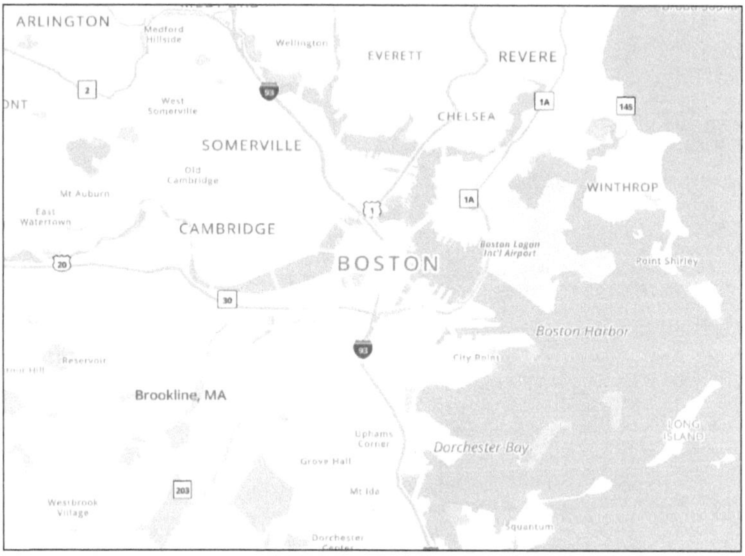

JFK was born in Brookline, Massachusetts, a suburb of Boston.

3. Sick Infancy: 1917–1920 (Ages 0-2)

Illness Hit Fast and Hard

Infancy is generally considered to be the first two years of life. JFK didn't wait long after his birth to initiate his strange medical saga. Infectious disease came early and hard by the time he was three months old. His mother kept a card file on JFK's childhood illnesses as well as her other eight children. During his infancy, he had multiple infections of his ears, nose, throat, and lungs. He nearly died when he was two years old. He came down with a severe case of scarlet fever which in that time period, often caused death, because penicillin and other antibiotics were not discovered until about two decades later. Scarlet fever was a complication of streptococcus tonsillitis and/or pharyngitis. The infection starts with a sore throat accompanied by chills, fever, vomiting, and tachycardia. Within about twenty-four hours red blotches appear on the skin. This strain of streptococcus would often cause hemorrhages in the red blotches as well as internal bleeding. JFK was in a local hospital and Maine sanitorium for two months and managed to survive.

At no time in JFK's infancy was he given any overall causative diagnosis for his multiple infections and symptoms. No connection to genetic tendencies was considered. Autoimmunity was a concept barely recognized even at the time of his death. Children were generally categorized by family and physicians as well or sickly. Childhood death was common as antibiotics were not developed until the World War II era. Only a few crude laboratory assays for anemia as well as diagnostic criteria for some infectious diseases had been developed. Rose Kennedy wrote in her memoir, "Jack was a very, very sick little boy."

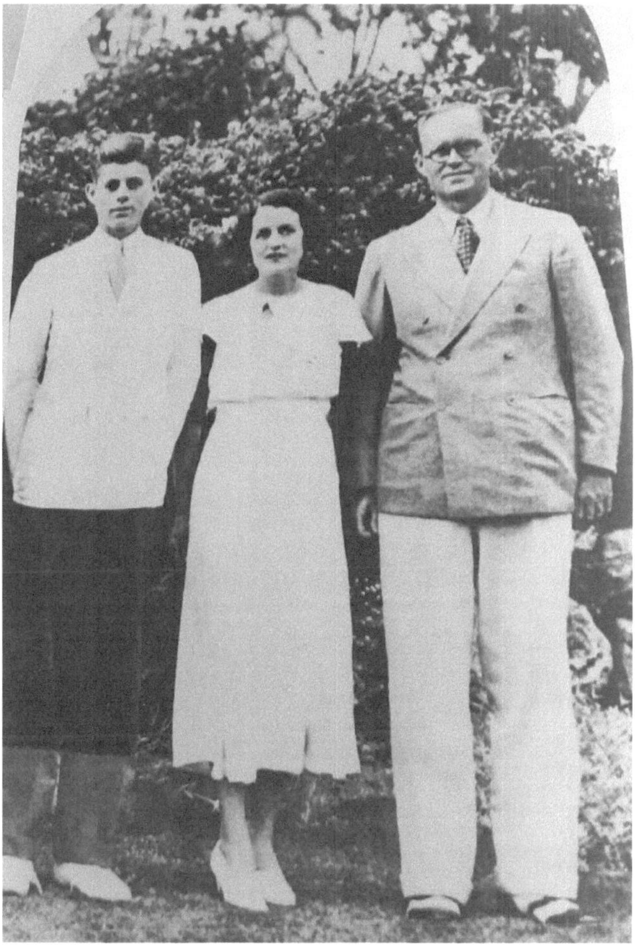

JFK with his mother, Rose and father, Joe.

4. Infectious Childhood: 1921–1930 (Ages 3-13)

No Infection Left Behind

Childhood is generally considered the time between the end of infancy at age two and puberty at about age thirteen. During 1927 the Kennedy family relocated to Riverdale, New York, and they also acquired a summer home in Hyannis Port, Massachusetts. JFK's childhood was characterized and highlighted by one infection after another. He was plagued by German measles, mumps, measles, whooping cough, chicken pox, bronchitis, and ear infections. He not only caught all the usual and expected childhood infections, but endured many others. Besides overt infections he continually complained of or experienced nausea, diarrhea, headache, and fatigue. He occasionally complained of joint pain. His incessant illnesses naturally caused the family great anxiety about his survival.

JFK suffered, as a youth, from many injuries and bruises sustained trying to achieve in sports where his physique was inadequate. He had a bizarre collision with his older brother,

Joe. Although Joe came away unscathed, JFK's wounds required twenty-eight stitches.

There is essentially no recording as to any specific medical care he received during his childhood. It is known that the Kennedy family had close contact with the best doctors in Boston at the time. There is little information, however, as to what medicinal substances and measures his physicians prescribed in the 1920's and 30's. Extracts from glands such as the adrenals and thyroid and some metals such as arsenic were commonly prescribed. Penicillin was not discovered until 1940. Whatever his physicians and family did to pull JFK through his infectious childhood will remain somewhat of a mystery. As a young boy, his mother remembered him as "bedridden and elfin-like."

Joan and Clay Blair in their book, "The Search for JFK" visited the Brookline Kennedy home and were able to copy down information from Rose Kennedy's card-file, which she kept on each of her children. She had carefully entered the dates; the illnesses and the age of her children when each became ill. The notes available to the Blair's on JFK are as follows:

February 20, 1920, age 2 ¾ years, scarlet fever, whooping cough, measles, and chicken pox.

Updated: City Hospital, Dr. Hill, Dr. Reardon, and took care of ear.

1928: German measles, Schick test, bronchitis occasionally.
June 15, 1930: Examined by Lahey clinic, tonsils, and adenoids OK.

October to December 1930: While at Canterbury, his weight fell from 99 ¾ to 99 ½ lbs.

December 31, 1930: Examined by Dr. Schloss. Good

condition. Loss of weight attributed to lack of milk in diet.

May 2, 1931: Appendicitis operation, surgery done by Dr. Verdie of New Haven. Performed at Danbury Hospital.

March 21, 1931: Glasses prescribed for reading by Dr. John Wheeler.

August 31, 1933: Tonsils and adenoids out-Dr. Kahill, St. Margaret's Hospital.

Now that we know he had a genetic, autoimmune, endocrine disorder, which is described in detail in later chapters, it is somewhat of a miracle that he survived childhood since his immune system was impaired at that time. Whatever and however he was treated be it medicinal, nutritional, spiritual, or all of the above, he somehow managed to pull through childhood.

5. Teenage Tragedies: 1931–1936 (Ages 14-19)

Gastrointestinal Disease Sets In

Puberty is the time in life that children undergo hormonal changes that result in physical and anatomic changes as well as emotional and sexual attitudes and desires. It usually begins at about age thirteen and ushers in what is called adolescence or the teenage years of thirteen to nineteen. The onset of puberty and adolescence changed Jack's pattern of illness from purely infectious to non-infectious maladies.

In 1930, at age thirteen, JFK was afflicted with an undiagnosed illness that restricted his activities. From October to December, he lost four to six pounds, felt "pretty tired, and did not grow. One doctor attributed it to a lack of milk in his diet, but that failed to explain why during a chapel service at the Canterbury School, his boarding school in New Milford, Connecticut, he felt "sick, dizzy, and weak." He wrote to his father, "I just about fainted, and everything began to get black, so I went out and then I fell, and Mr. Hume (the headmaster) caught me. I am O.K. now." In April of 1931 JFK collapsed with abdominal pains, and the surgeon who examined him concluded that it was appendicitis and that an operation was necessary at the nearby hospital in Danbury, Connecticut.

The operation did not solve the problem. In the fall of 1932, after transferring to another boarding school called Choate School, in Wallingford, Connecticut, JFK complained of abdominal discomfort and fatigue. His weight was only 117 pounds which was less than robust for a fifteen-year-old-boy. In January and February 1933 "flu-like symptoms" plagued him, along with periodic pain in his knees.

"Jack's winter term sounded like a hospital report," a school official recounted at the fiftieth anniversary of his attendance at Choate. There was correspondence flying back and forth between Rose Kennedy and the headmaster's wife. "Again, it seemed like his eyes, ears, teeth, knees, arches, from the top of his head to the tip of his toes, all needed attention."

At about age 15, JFK experienced joint pains, particularly in his knees. Little did anyone know or expect that these joint symptoms were a component to a generalized, genetic, autoimmune disorder that would eventually cause dysfunction and impairments throughout his entire body.

Over the summer of 1933, he gained no weight. Matters got worse the following year. In the winter of 1934, he became very sick and had to be rushed by ambulance to New Haven Hospital for observation. His symptoms included weight loss and a bad case of hives. Doctors feared that he had leukemia and began regularly checking his blood counts.

In June of 1934, as his junior year at Choate ended, he began feeling ill again. His major symptoms were related to his gastrointestinal tract that included pain, bloating, diarrhea, and vomiting. His parents sent him to the famous Mayo Clinic, in

Rochester, Minnesota. He spent a miserable month there. He wrote to his best and life-long friend, Lem Billings, "the God-damnest hole I've ever seen." He was initially hospitalized at Mayo but transferred to nearby St. Mary's Hospital after two weeks. He helped maintain his sanity and kept up his hopes for a return to friends and family through a series of letters to them. JFK handled what he feared was a life-threatening disease with a biting wit and a refusal to complain openly to anyone but his close friends. Judging from the medical tests described in the correspondence and in later medical records, JFK had colitis, which was initially thought to be peptic-ulcer disease. The doctors began by prescribing a diet of bland food preparatory to tests that he had hoped would be over in a few days. But the exams lasted much longer. "I am suffering terribly out here," he wrote to Lem Billings. "*I now have a gut ache all the time. I'm still eating peas and corn for my food.*" He expected to be there for at least another twelve days. Two days later he wrote Lem, "*God what a beating I'm taking. I've lost 8 lbs. And still going down…I'm showing them a thing or two. Nobody able to figure what's wrong with me. All they do is talk about what an interesting case.*"

All the gastrointestinal and colon tests indicated that JFK had colitis and digestive problems, which made it difficult for him to gain weight and threatened deadly consequences if the colon became ulcerated or bled.

Judging from accounts published in the January 1934 and December 1936 issues of the Mayo Clinic Journal Proceedings, the clinic's usual therapy for colitis involved a combination of restricted diet and relief of emotional stress, which was assumed to be a major contributor to both colitis and ulcers; and injections of serum obtained from horses. Although the clinic claimed a measure of success with this treatment, it was clearly no panacea. JFK was probably given adrenal gland extracts which research centers were then testing. It seemed promising for the treatment of a whole variety of illnesses.[2,5,13,28]

From September of 1934 to June of 1935, at ages 16 and 17, JFK's senior year of prep school, the school infirmary kept a close watch on his blood count. Joe Kennedy passed these records on to the Mayo doctors. At that time there was concern that JFK might be suffering from leukemia. In retrospect, any changes in his blood count may have been a reaction to the drugs he was taking. When he fell ill the following autumn, a doctor advised that he had agranulocytosis, a decrease in granular white blood cells, which made him more susceptible to infections.

Shortly after leaving Choate Prep School, JFK had to spend two months at the Peter Bent Brigham Hospital, in Boston. Uncertain whether they were dealing strictly with colitis or with a combination of colitis and ulcers, they worried that his medicines were playing havoc with his white-blood-cell count. Consequently, his doctors performed additional tests. According to a letter he wrote to Lem Billings, his white-blood-cell count was 6,000 when he entered the hospital and down to 3,500 three weeks later. "At 1500 you die," JFK joked. "They call me 2000 to go Kennedy." Fortunately, this issue resolved itself.

Although JFK began having joint pain and experienced a low white blood cell count, his teenage years were primarily that of gastrointestinal disease and its attendant disability. Today, he would undoubtedly be given a diagnosis of "celiac disease" or "irritable bowel syndrome" rather than the diagnoses of "duodenitis" or "spastic colon." The term celiac is derived from the Greek word "koilia" which means a "hallow" or "cavity." Today, celiac disease is generally believed to be an autoimmune disorder with gluten insensitivity.[2,23] Regardless of terminology, JFK experienced gastrointestinal symptoms throughout his entire life.

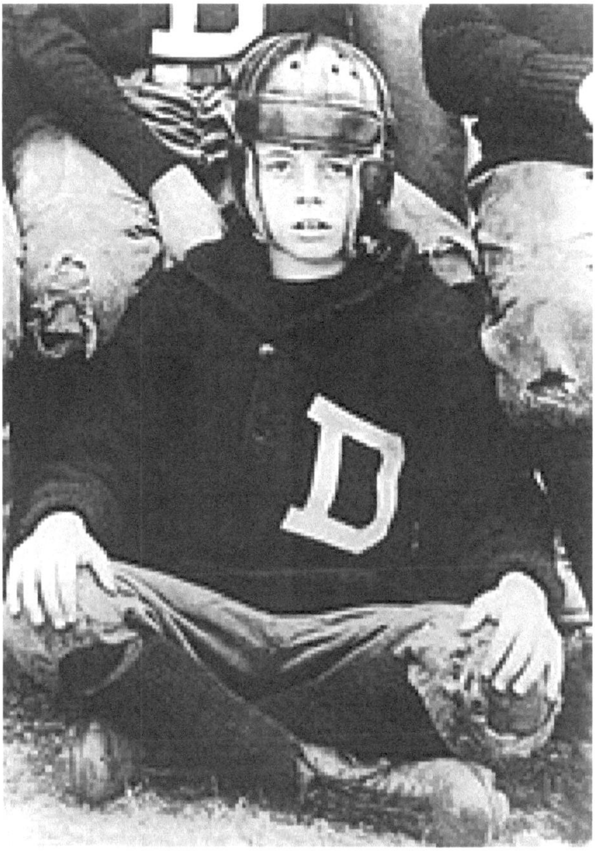

JFK was quite athletic despite his genetic diseases, but he did not recover well from injuries and bruises.

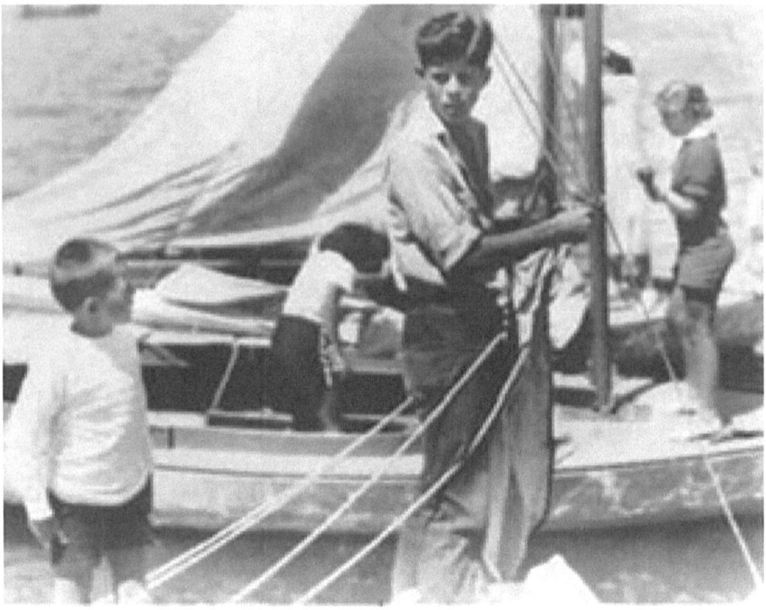

JFK was thin as a teenager. His gastrointestinal disease prohibited weight gain.

6. College Calamities: 1936–1940 (Ages 19-23)

The Pain Begins

JFK's gastrointestinal issues sufficiently resolved by the Fall of 1936 to enroll in Harvard University. Therefore, he was able to enroll in Harvard University, at age 19. At this time, he was six feet tall and weighed 147 pounds.

Disregarding his recurring list of health problems and being underweight, Jack tried out for the football team as a freshman. Not surprisingly, during a practice session he injured his "unstable back" and had to be carried from the practice field in great pain. This injury was the initiation of his significant and devastating pain problem that lasted his entire life.

He recovered from the football back injury and tried out for the swimming team. This venture also ended in frustration. He developed a flu-like illness which kept him in the college infirmary for a month.

He was doing well enough by summer break, however, in 1937 to travel to Europe. Without warning, he developed hives, swelling, and an episode of a low white blood cell count. In early 1938 at age 21, his gastrointestinal problems returned and lasted for about two years before a remission occurred. This recurrence was preceded by two hospitalizations and more visits to the Mayo Clinic. In February of 1938 he first went back to the Mayo Clinic for more studies, but with no good results. In June he spent two weeks in New England Baptist Hospital for the same complaints, but again experienced no improvement. In October he was still "in rotten shape," but he refused to re-enter the hospital for more of what now seemed like pointless tests. In February of 1939, however, he gave in and went back to the Mayo Clinic. It was the same old routine: a diet of bland foods three times a day and another proctoscopy of his colon. By November, he was under the care of Dr. William Murphy, of Harvard, the physician and Nobel laureate who co-discovered the treatment for pernicious anemia and had an uncommon faith in the healing power of liver extracts. Jack recorded that he was going to "take my first liver injection today and I hope they work." They did not.

Robert Dallek, in his JFK health monograph in the 2002 "Atlantic" and his brilliant book, "An Unfinished Life: John F. Kennedy," believed JFK may have been started on deoxycorticosterone (DOCA) for his gastrointestinal disorder. DOCA had just recently been invented.[5] It was a small pellet that was implanted under the skin. This possibility is discussed, in detail, in a later chapter. Regardless, a year later he was still wrestling with abdominal pain, spastic colon, and low weight. In fact, some of these symptoms continued to plague him throughout life.

While at Harvard in 1938, he began having occasional pains in his right sacroiliac joint. It apparently grew worse but at times he was completely free from symptoms. In the latter part of 1940 while playing tennis he experienced a sudden pain in his lower right back-it seemed to him that "something had slipped." He was hospitalized at the Lahey Clinic for ten days. A low back support was applied, and he was comfortable. Since that time, he had periodic attacks of a similar nature. It is unclear if he was started on any chronic medication for his back.

Despite his on-going health issues in college, he graduated from Harvard in 1939 at age 22. Along the way he published his thesis which became a book entitled "Why England Slept." Shortly after graduating he returned to the Mayo Clinic for a check-up and was advised to take a year-long leave to recuperate from his illness. JFK did not take this advice and enrolled in the Stanford School of Business. He again fell ill, withdrew, and returned to the Lahey Clinic in Boston in 1941, at which time he was again hospitalized at the New England Baptist Hospital. He was treated for recurrences of gastrointestinal distress, fever, weakness, and back pain. No precise details of this hospitalization have been publicized but he recovered to the point that he desired to enter military service.

JFK's college years at Harvard and Stanford were filled with calamitics. His gastrointestinal problems would only calm down for short periods, and he began his long career of devastating back pain. It is remarkable that he was able to graduate and even publish a book.

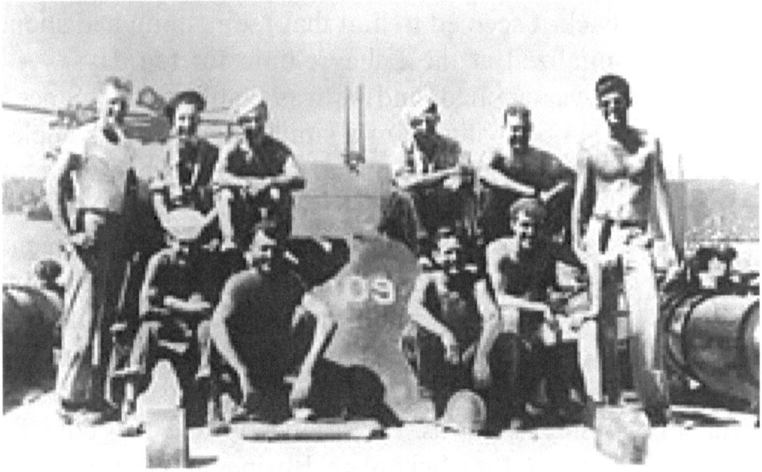

He remained tall and thin throughout life. Pictured here is his PT109 crew, 1943.

7. The PT109 Incident: 1941–1945 (Ages 24-28)

Lucky to Survive

After graduating from Harvard in 1940, at age 23, he had a checkup at Mayo and traveled to Latin America with his mother and sister, Eunice. He then registered at Stanford University School of Business. While he was still at Stanford, he registered for the draft on October 16, 1940. He was officially drafted on October 29, 1940, but as a student at Stanford, he could defer until July 1941. In the summer of 1941, he volunteered for the Army Officers Candidate School. He failed the physical, presumably because of his bad back. He then tried to enlist in the Navy, which at that time failed to pass him. He reapplied and was commissioned as an ensign in the US Naval Reserve on September 25, 1941. It has been reported that JFK used powerful influence-namely his father-to accomplish this.

Within months JFK's back trouble began to erupt, but he recovered and was declared fit for military duty in June 1942.

He had applied for and been accepted into midshipmen's school in the Spring of 1942 with an eye on sea duty. He was ultimately accepted to patrol torpedo (PT) boat training school. This was a highly competitive position, and some biographers believe his prominent father had to again use his influence to get Jack's admission to the school. JFK finished his PT boat training and was ordered to the Pacific theater on January 8, 1943.

In August 1943 JFK endured his famous PT109 incident. His boat became involved in an action in Blackett Strait, between two islands in the Solomon Islands. A Japanese destroyer rammed JFK's boat and destroyed it. Two crew members were killed. JFK and the rest of the crew were stranded. JFK reportedly towed a badly wounded crewman with the strap of his life jacket clenched between his teeth for a three to five hours swim to a nearby island where he and his crew were eventually rescued.

While assigned to PT109, his back problems were recorded by Lennie Thom, JFK's executive officer. He wrote letters home discussing JFK's back problem and his refusal to report to sick bay. "Jack feigned being well. He did not let on to his crew or his commanding officer that he was ill or in pain. He couldn't, however, hide his chronic back ailment since he always wore a corset-type brace and kept a plywood board under his mattress." Although it is often assumed that JFK's back problems began with this heroic event, it, in fact, worsened his already diseased back.

JFK was assigned to a second PT boat, the PT59, a few weeks after PT109. The new PT boat was converted to a gunboat. As usual, however, his recurrent bouts of gastrointestinal pain, nausea, and diarrhea hit him shortly after his second PT boat assignment. On November 18, 1943 he was medically directed to leave PT59 and be hospitalized. He was believed to have contracted malaria which was very common among sailors in the Pacific theater. He left the South Pacific before Christmas on military leave. A friend in Los Angeles described him as looking "ghastly, thin, and drawn."

His request to transfer to the mainland was approved in January 1944. He was later to be honorably discharged in November 1944 for a disability primarily related to his back. He received the Navy and Marine Corp Medal on June 12, 1944, just prior to his first major surgery on June 23, 1944.

Although the general public may believe that the PT109 incident caused JFK's back problem, it actually accelerated and worsened his already diseased spine. It is possible that if the PT109 incident had not occurred that his lifetime of misery and back surgery would not have occurred. Besides worsening of his back, JFK had to continuously fight his never-ending colitis. To top it off, he had to survive a bout of malaria.

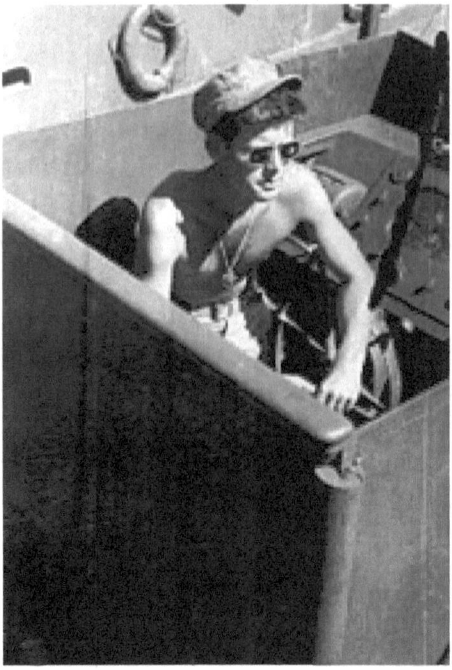

Kennedy on his Navy patrol boat, PT-109, 1943

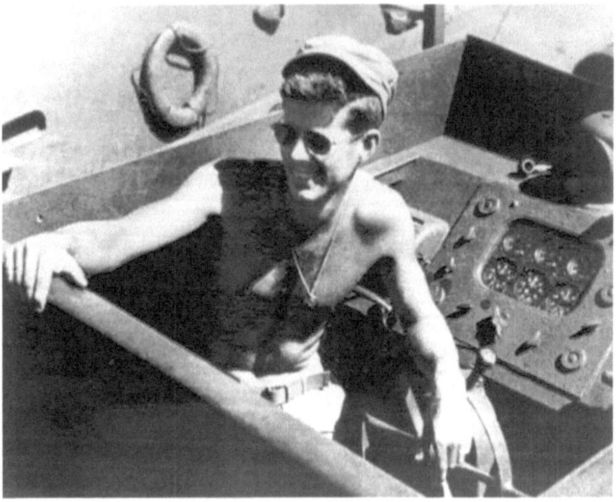

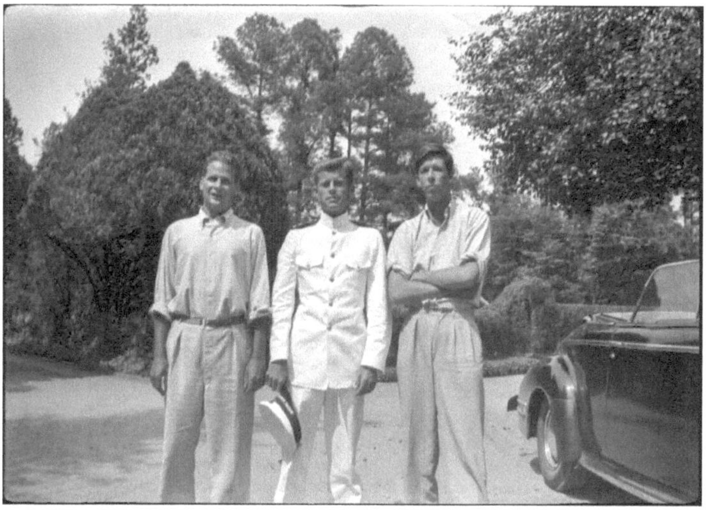

John F. Kennedy (wearing his United States Navy officer's dress white uniform and holding his U.S. Navy cap) poses beside a car with family friends, John "Zeke" Coleman, Jr. (left), and Charles "Chuck" Spalding, in Charleston, South Carolina.

8. First Failed Back Surgery: June 23, 1944 (Age 27)

Mysterious Non-Improvement

Jack continued to be plagued with back pain after graduating from Harvard University in June 1940. He was referred to Dr. Gilbert "Ned" Haggart, an orthopedic spine specialist at the Lahey Clinic in Boston, who diagnosed him with a "very unstable lumbosacral joint." Dr. Haggart recommended a course of conservative treatment in the form of manipulation of the back under anesthesia, which JFK underwent at the Lahey Clinic in 1940. Dr. Haggart also introduced the idea of sacroiliac fusion if the non-surgical measures failed. He later suffered a back pain flare while doing calisthenics in March 1942. He was hospitalized twice for sacroiliac and back pain.

The collision of PT109 with the Japanese destroyer in late 1943 and the enduring and grueling nature of the subsequent rescue worsened JFK's back problems. Once he returned stateside, he was evaluated by a team of physicians at the Mayo Clinic, including noted orthopedist Dr. Ralph Gormley, who summarized Lt. Kennedy's condition at that time as "confined...to the region of the left sacroiliac with pain in the posterior part of the left hip down as far as the knee."

Given that JFK's presentation was not an obvious one for a herniated disc, he underwent an air myelogram, and the Mayo team stated that "a diagnosis of a protruded disc was not defined...at this time you are not in need of surgery." He may possibly have had a myelogram with Pantopaque® dye as an x-ray taken later by the British physician Dr. Daniel Davis, in 1947, showed residue of the dye in his spinal canal.

Kennedy eventually proceeded with surgery. He was admitted to New England Baptist Hospital, and on June 23, 1944, he underwent a left lumbar 4 and 5 laminectomy and lumbar 5 to S1 discectomy performed by Dr. James Poppen, neurosurgeon at the Lahey Clinic. JFK did well for two weeks postoperatively, before the onset of severe muscle spasms which occurred when he attempted to ambulate. At six weeks postoperatively, however, Dr. Poppen wrote:

"On June twenty-third I did a unilateral exploration of the fourth and fifth lumbar interspaces. The fourth space was completely normal. However, the nerve in the fifth interspace was reddened and underlying this, the disc interspace material was abnormally soft, and the posterior longitudinal ligament was firmly adherent to the nerve root. There, however, was very little protrusion of the ruptured cartilage. A thorough removal of the degenerative portion of the cartilage was carried out...The patient did well following the operation for a period of two weeks. Upon having the patient get up and about, however, severe muscle spasm in the low back took place. This necessitated fairly large doses of narcotics to keep him comfortable...I have had no other patients in a series of over five hundred ruptured intervertebral discs with a similar experience...I am indeed sorry that this had to happen with Lieutenant Kennedy."

This account shows that the surgeon in charge was mystified at the poor outcome of surgery. Years later, after his death, some experts believe he may have developed a complication, even possibly before the surgery, known as adhesive arachnoiditis. This disease involves only spinal cord nerve roots that are inside the spinal canal. Surgery involving the discs would not, therefore, benefit him and likely made him worse. Regardless of the cause of surgical failure, JFK was subsequently transferred to the Chelsea Naval Hospital for recovery and another evaluation. JFK was described as "obviously incapacitated by pain in the low back and down the left leg." JFK realized that the surgery had done little good. He wrote to a friend, "the doc should have read just one more book before picking up the saw."

While recovering at Chelsea Naval Hospital in the fall of 1944, JFK received word that his older brother, Joe, had been killed in action in England. Late in 1944, JFK's back troubles eventually eased up although his gastrointestinal difficulties continued. Given his recalcitrant medical issues, the Navy declared him permanently unfit for service on November 25, 1944. JFK was back in the civilian sector, now the heir to the family's political aspirations since his brother had died and who the family believed had great political potential. Since his surgery did not relieve his pain, he continued to wear his corset and practice any other respite he could muster. To a great extent he appeared to accept his plight and go on with his life.

9. Addison's Disease and Cortisone: 1946–1950 (Ages 29-33)

Last Rites and Controversy

Dr. Thomas Addison, in 1855, published a monogram entitled, "On the Constitutional and Local Effects of Disease of the Supra-Renal Capsules." At this time in history, the glands that sit on top of each kidney were called "supra-renal capsules." because they were encased in a capsule-like covering. For short, the name adrenal, meaning "on top the kidneys." was later adopted. Dr. Addison presented both the clinical history, symptoms, and autopsy findings of eleven cases. At autopsy the adrenals of his subjects were mainly infiltrated with cancer, syphilis, or tuberculosis.

In life, some of the cases had severe pain and at autopsy had a matted and inflamed cauda equina, which would probably be called adhesive arachnoiditis in today's medical world. The attached table is a summary of major clinical symptoms of what is now called Addison's disease.

Characteristics of Addison's Disease

(The disease today is confirmed by low blood cortisone levels)

Anorexia (loss of appetite)

Black freckles on head or neck

Bronze skin

Bluish pigmentation in mouth

Hypotension (low blood pressure)

Fatigue

Hypoglycemia (low blood sugar)

Vomiting

Weakness

Weight loss

JFK, in retrospect, fits Dr. Addison's original description of the disease. It was primarily in males between the ages of twenty and sixty usually commencing insidiously and proceeding very slowly so as to occur over a period ranging from several weeks to even months or years. In a lecture to the South London Medical Society in 1849, Dr Addison described his findings even before he published his enduring monograph.[1,3] A short excerpt of his lecture is given here as it describes a great deal about JFK and his strange medical saga.

> *"It usually occurs between the ages of 20 and 60; sometimes proceeding to an extreme degree in a few weeks, but more frequently weeks, or even months, before any very serious alarm is taken either by the patient or by the patient's friends. Its approach is first indicated by a certain amount of languor and muscular strength, general relaxation or feebleness of the whole frame, and indisposition to, or incapacity for, bodily or mental exertion. These symptoms go on increasing with greater or less rapidity: the face, lips, conjunctive, and external surface of the body, become more and more bloodless; the tongue appears pale and flabby; the heart's action gets exceedingly enfeebled, with a weak, soft, unusually large, but always strikingly compressible pulse; the appetite may or may not be lost; the patient experiences a distressing and increasing sense of helplessness and faintness; the heart is excited, or rendered tumultuous in its action, the breathing painfully hurried by the slightest exertion, whilst the whole surface bears some resemblance to a bad wax figure: the patient is no longer able to rise from his bed; slight edema perhaps shows itself about the ankles; the feeling of faintness and weakness becomes extreme, and he dies either from sheer exhaustion, or death is preceded by signs of passive effusion or cerebral compression."*

Note that in the short excerpt by Dr. Addison he mentions some of JFK's medical issues. He had anemia and his skin was even called "yellow" or "bronze" by some observers. He was plagued throughout life with stomach irritability.[23]

JFK's Addison's disease was diagnosed in 1947 by a renowned British physician, Sir Daniel Davis. He was age thirty at the time. JFK exhibited some classic Addison symptoms and characteristics of this disease in the two years prior to this diagnosis. As stated by Dr. Addison, the disease is insidious and slowly progressive.

The Navy declared JFK permanently unfit for service on November 25, 1944. Shortly after his discharge in March 1945, he returned to the Mayo Clinic but didn't stay long. He went to Castle Hot Springs, Arizona, in an attempt to recover his health. It was an elusive quest as his back pain and colitis symptoms didn't resolve. Consequently, a month later (May 1945) his pain somewhat subsided enough to take a job as a correspondent for the Hearst Newspapers. His travel assignments included San Francisco, Great Britain, and Germany.

In April 1946, JFK declared his candidacy for the US House of Representatives, Massachusetts 11th district. The next several months of campaigning exhausted the 29-year-old JFK. One campaign worker declared him to be "crippled." His back pain returned, and he required a daily regimen of therapy involving back rubs, hot baths, and regular use of his back brace. The rigors of campaigning took their toll, culminating with JFK's collapse while marching in the Annual Bunker Hill Parade on June 17, 1946. He walked the entire five miles through Charleston, Massachusetts on the hot and sunny day and collapsed at the end. This occurred 24 hours before the election. Nonetheless, the following day JFK was elected to Congress.

During the campaign he weighed only 150 pounds and looked quite frail on his six-foot frame. As the campaign progressed, aids said he seemed tired, hollow-eyed, and anemic looking. Witnesses who saw JFK collapse after the parade say he turned "very yellow and blue." After JFK took office, he didn't "slow down and smell any roses." He took an eventful trip to England in 1947, his first year in office. While there he collapsed and was hospitalized. Sir Daniel Davis, the admitting physician, diagnosed adrenal failure or Addison's disease. He told JFK's close friend, Pamela Churchill, "that American friend of yours, he hasn't got a year to live." Although there is no known specific reason as to why Dr. Davis believed this to be the case, he must have read Dr. Addison's original monograph in which the subjects died within months after symptoms set in. He obviously made the diagnosis of Addison's strictly on the presence of multiple clinical characteristics.

It is not known what treatments Dr. Davis may have rendered. Dr. Davis likely gave him a cortisone derivative called deoxycorticosterone acetate (DOCA) which was the only treatment at that time. JFK recovered enough, however, in London to make it back to the USA by sailing on the Queen Mary. He was accompanied by a nurse and was then admitted to the Lahey Clinic in Boston. His condition was considered so serious that a priest was brought on board when the ship docked in New York to read his last rites of the Catholic Church. He was carried off the ship on a stretcher, flown to Boston, and hospitalized at the Lahey Clinic. He was stabilized and left the hospital continuing to maintain on DOCA. This tablet was implanted under the skin. Whether or not he used DOCA prior to his trip to England is uncertain, but his possible prior use is described below. Although the dosage and frequency of his DOCA skin implantations in 1947 is unknown, he was stabilized well enough to carry out a vigorous effort to advance his political career. Over the five-year period between 1947 and 1952 he kept up a vigorous schedule. To bolster his statewide profile, Congressman Kennedy began crisscrossing Massachusetts, usually beginning at dawn and ending after midnight – an intense schedule likely to have aggravated and worsened his back condition. Dave Powers, his longtime political adviser, stated that JFK had to travel "with crutches-gritting his teeth when he walked-but then when he came into the room where the crowd was gathered, he was erect and smiling. He looked as fit and healthy as the light-heavyweight champion of the world. Then after he finished his speech, answered questions from the floor, and shook hands with everyone, we would help him into the car, and he would lean back on the seat and close his eyes in pain." His grueling schedule and hard work seemed to pay off. After seven years in the House of Representatives, JFK was elected to the US Senate in 1952.

After JFK's formal diagnosis of Addison's in 1947, his physicians appeared to manage his adrenal insufficiency with considerable expertise. At no time until his death is there any record that he had an adrenal crisis as he did in London in 1947. His health issues shifted almost exclusively to his back pain. It became progressively worse and so disabling that he chose in October, 1954 to undergo a double fusion, metal implant procedure, on his lumbar-sacral spine.

Between 1947 and 1955 Dr. Ephraim Shorr, an endocrinologist at New York Hospital, took over JFK's adrenal care. During his major spine surgery in 1954, Dr. Shorr supervised his endocrine needs. At this time, there was considerable fear about performing surgery on a patient with Addison's disease. Severe trauma and stress that accompany major surgery requires increased adrenal output of cortisone and other hormones. Little did the physicians involved in the surgery know that their prominent patient, JFK, would later become an icon to the world. After the surgery, they published a paper involving JFK's case. The paper was in the July 1955 issue of the "Archives of Surgery." and it was entitled, "The Management of Adrenal Cortical Insufficiency During Surgery."[22] Without naming JFK, they described a 37-year-old male with a seven-year history of Addison's disease. They noted he had a DOCA implant of 150 mg every three months and was taking cortisone 25 mg by mouth on a daily basis. These dosages indicate total hormone replacement due to adrenals that were hardly functioning. It is unknown, however, just how long he had taken cortisone. This extract of the adrenal glands was discovered and originally called "compound E" in 1949. The first use of cortisone was in patients with rheumatoid arthritis who responded extremely well to this new treatment. Additional studies showed that the adrenal glands produce about 25 to 30 mg of cortisone a day. Dr. Shorr started JFK on cortisone shortly after it was discovered and maintained JFK well enough to get him through his major surgery which is described in more detail in a later chapter.

Fortunately, JFK lived through the surgery, but he developed severe post-surgical complications. The surgical site didn't heal, became infected, and required removal of an implanted metal plate, antibiotics, and wound debridement. He was post-operatively given "last rites" a second time, but again managed to survive. In summary, JFK is a great example of complications that can occur in a person with Addison's who requires surgery or sustains some other severe stress and needs extra cortisone to carry them through the event.

JFK's Addison's Disease continued to be well-managed after the surgery. Dr. Eugene Cohen became JFK's endocrinologist in 1957 after the retirement of Dr. Shorr.

Dr. Lee Mandel, a US Naval endocrinologist, in 2008, analyzed JFK's records maintained at the John F. Kennedy Presidential Library and Museum. He expertly determined that JFK's Addison's disease was a component of a rare, genetic disease called "autoimmune polyglandular disease." Autoimmunity, described in later chapters, is an intrinsic biologic disorder that attacks and destroys tissues over time (e.g., automatic "rusting" of tissues). In JFK's case this included not only his adrenals, but thyroid, intestine, testicles, joints, and spine. In Dr. Mandel's analysis of JFK, he found that in October 1961, he was taking cortisone 10 mg daily, prednisone 2.5 mg twice daily, and fludrocortisone 0.1 mg daily. Vitamin C, which is involved in adrenal metabolism, was taken in a 500 mg dose twice daily (mg is milligram). This program, even by today's standards, could be considered exceptional. In addition to adrenal gland hormonal replacement, he required thyroid and testicular hormones. JFK's overall health progressively improved beginning when Drs Janet Travell and Cohen took over his case after his failed surgery in 1954. In the late 1950's there were multiple hospitalizations, but steady improvement carried forward until his death in 1963.

JFK's use of cortisone derivatives prior to his diagnosis of Addison's disease in 1947 may have occurred. In fact, the use of cortisone derivatives may well have saved him during his early years.

In 2002, Robert Dallek, a renowned historian, and his medical consultant, Dr. Jeffrey Kelman, were the first researchers to be allowed to review medical records in the John F. Kennedy Presidential Library and Museum. Mr. Dallek published his medical findings in "The Atlantic" in December 2002, in an article entitled "The Medical Ordeals of JFK." These researchers came to the conclusion that JFK had taken the cortisone derivative, DOCA, prior to his diagnosis of Addison's in 1947.

At some point between Addison's report in 1855 and the end of the 19th century, physicians began to treat Addison's disease by administering whole adrenal gland extracts from animals, mainly cattle, that had gone to slaughter. This practice was known as "organotherapy."[12,28] This treatment including whole, dried adrenal glands, were also given for symptomatic treatment of a wide variety of diseases as few disease-specific medications were available in the 1930's.

A historical review of JFK's health issues clearly suggests that he had periodic episodes of low production of cortisone. These episodes probably aggravated his gastrointestinal symptoms and infections beginning in childhood. Within a few weeks after his birth, JFK started having incessant infections. He almost died due to scarlet fever before age three. His susceptibility to infections in childhood was clearly in excess compared to normal children. A healthy adrenal gland carries a stored reserve of cortisone and other hormones to ward off infections. Between ages 10 and 15 he developed gastrointestinal disease which plagued him all his life. The genetic autoimmune disease that progressively destroyed his adrenal glands also attacked his stomach and intestine and created periodic symptoms of nausea, bloating, diarrhea, bleeding, pain, and inability to gain weight. Other manifestations that are recognized as autoimmune and aggravated by low cortisone include joint pains and osteoporosis. [20,23,37,38]

Mr. Dallek in his Atlantic article and in his extensive JFK biography, "An Unfinished Life," stated that he believed JFK started on DOCA when it was synthetically produced in 1937. This is probably a fact because his physicians had probably found that whole adrenal gland administration and/or DOCA, itself, relieved many of his gastrointestinal and arthritic symptoms. They did not suspect Addison's disease. For example, when JFK was 23 years old, he went to Mayo Clinic for his gastrointestinal disorder, and they found he had low blood pressure which is a rather constant finding in Addison's. Dr. Paul O'Leary of Mayo Clinic described JFK's situation in a letter to JFK's father in August 1940: *"Jack's examination revealed a rather unique finding which he perhaps discussed with you by this time. His blood pressure was exceedingly low, being in the neighborhood of 85, and for a boy his age (23 years) it should be approximately 120. This so-called static hypotension is a comparatively recently recognized entity, and it might well be that some of Jack's gastrointestinal difficulties are attributable to this finding."* It is notable that Dr. O'Leary discusses hypotension and gastrointestinal issues in his letter but doesn't mention adrenal glands or Addison's. Given the thoroughness of the Mayo Clinic in those years the letter would undoubtedly have mentioned Addison's if it was suspected.

Mr. Dallek's belief that JFK was started on DOCA in 1937 is well grounded. DOCA was made as a tablet that had to be implanted under the skin. In early 1937, in a handwritten note from JFK to his father, Jack worried about getting a prescription filled in Cambridge, Massachusetts, where he was a freshman at Harvard College. "*Ordering stuff here very (illegible word). I would be sure you get the prescriptions. Some of the stuff as it is very potent, and he (Jack's doctor) seems to be keeping it pretty quiet.*"

Given that cortisone medication, either as an adrenal extract or by a tablet of DOCA implanted under the skin, it is reasonable to assume that the prescription was for one of these two adrenal treatment agents. Moreover, nine years later in 1946 and before he received the diagnosis of Addison's disease in 1947, JFK's friend, Paul Fay, watched him implant a pellet of DOCA in his leg.[22] Fay remembered that Jack used a little knife to just barely cut the surface of the skin, try not to get blood, and then get underneath and put the tablet in and put a bandage over it. After the insertion Jack said, "hopefully this tablet would dissolve by the heat of the body and be absorbed by the bloodstream."

Mr. Dallek believed that JFK could have used excess DOCA and developed osteoporosis from it before JFK's surgery in 1944. Medical records, not x-rays, state the surgeons during JFK's 1944 spine surgery removed "some abnormally soft disc interspace material." It is now known that autoimmune diseases can cause deterioration of intervertebral discs. Since JFK's 1944 surgical records specifies that disc material rather than bone was removed. It is uncertain whether osteoporosis was present because x-rays taken at that time did not show it.[23] Relatively recent studies show that Addison's itself may cause osteoporosis and JFK appeared to have significant bone deterioration in later years .[38,39]

There is no hard evidence that JFK ever took corticosteroids in excess amounts. Excess amounts, produce a typical "cushingoid" picture named after Dr. Harvey Cushing, who described persons who have excess cortisone in the blood. These persons gain weight, have a rounded ("moon") face, purplish skin lines ("striae") and hypertension. JFK at no time demonstrated the tell-tale signs of excess cortisone.

In 1955 JFK demonstrated another condition described by Dr. Addison some 100 years prior. In 1849 he found that persons with adrenal destruction also had severe anemia. He called the anemia "pernicious" since it appeared highly destructive and fatal. Dr. Janet Travell, shortly after she took charge of JFK's medical care in 1955, found that JFK had pernicious anemia. It is now known to be caused by a vitamin B_{12} deficiency. Addison's disease has always been highly linked to anemia. For example, the Gould Medical Dictionary (6th Edition) in 1913 called "pernicious" anemia "Addison's Anemia." Also, in the early part of the last century, tuberculosis was the most common cause of Addison's. The 1913 Gould's Dictionary defined Addison's Disease as *"bronzed skin disease, caused by changes (especially tuberculosis) in the suprarenal capsules and neighboring sympathetic plexuses."* This association of tuberculosis and Addison's would later haunt JFK when he ran for President.

In summary, JFK appeared to have intermittent cortisone deficiency. He was lucky to survive his many severe infections. His doctors, in the 1930's, likely used whole adrenal gland extracts and/or the synthetic, weak cortisone derivative called DOCA to relieve his gastrointestinal symptoms. He was diagnosed with Addison's disease by the British physician, Dr. Daniel Davis, in 1947. He was so ill at this time that he was given "last rites" but managed to survive with the use of DOCA. Dr. Ephraim Shorr became JFK's endocrinologist in the late 1940's and started him on cortisone which he would take the rest of his life.

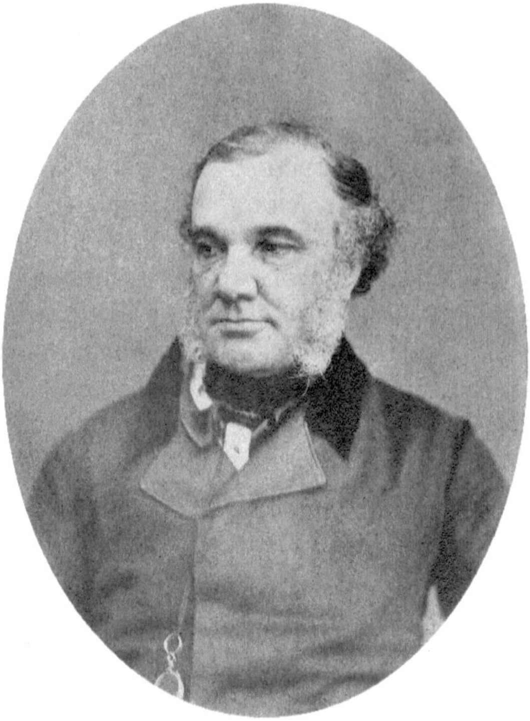

Dr. Thomas Addison in 1855 published a monograph on his discovery of adrenal failure and its clinical manifestations.

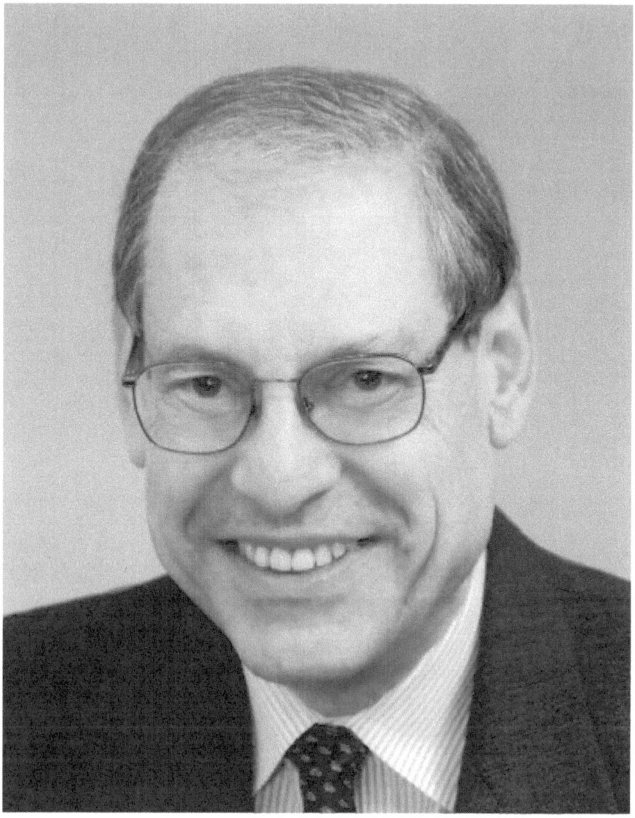

Famed historian, Robert Dallek, was the first to review JFK's medical records, and he produced a seminal report on his medical history.

10. Pain, Death Wish, and Failed Surgery: 1951-1954 (Age 34-37)

Last Rites Given a Second Time

Cortisone was discovered around 1950. Despite being started and maintained on it, along with DOCA, his back pain became progressively worse. It was constant. X-rays in Dr. Janet Travell's records showed that the fourth lumbar intervertebral space had narrowed. Her records stated there was a compression fracture and collapse of the fifth lumbar vertebrae. Apparently, his autoimmune disease had produced some osteoporosis.[38,39] JFK often needed crutches to get up a flight of stairs in the early 1950's.

In 1951 he took an around the world trip with his brother, Robert. When they reached Okinawa, Japan, JFK apparently came down with a severe infection and his temperature shot up to 106°. He entered a hospital in Okinawa where his doctors feared for his life. His doctors at the Lahey Clinic in Boston, however, prescribed by telephone extra dosages of cortisone and antibiotics. Miraculously, he again recovered from a near death experience. There is some belief that this crisis may have been precipitated by JFK failing to take his daily cortisone which he required to maintain adrenal function.

In 1952 during a successful campaign to replace Henry Cabot Lodge as senator from Massachusetts, JFK suffered headaches, upper respiratory infections, stomach aches, urinary tract discomfort, and nearly unceasing back pain. He consulted an ear, nose and throat specialist about his headaches; took anti-spasmodics and applied heat fifteen minutes a day to ease his stomach troubles; consulted urologists about his bladder and prostate discomfort; had DOCA pellets implanted and took daily oral doses of cortisone to control his Addison's disease. He constantly struggled to find even a little relief from his back pain.

Dave Powers, one of Kennedy's aides, remembers that at the end of each day on the road during the campaign, JFK would climb into the back seat of the car, where "he would lean back…and close his eyes in pain." At the hotel he would use crutches to get himself upstairs and then soak in a hot bath for an hour before going to bed. "The pain," Powers adds, "often made him tense and irritable with his fellow travelers."

On September 12, 1953, JFK married Jacqueline Bouvier. This author has not been able to identify any expectations, fears, or hopes of either party about JFK's health prior to their marriage. Sometimes a marriage partner, falsely but truly, believes that marriage can solve a health problem. Despite Jack and Jackie's marriage, by the Spring of 1954, Jack's back pain had become almost unbearable. He could not bend to pull a sock onto his left foot, and he had to ascend and descend stairs moving sideways. Beginning in May, he had to rely on crutches more than ever. Walks from his office to the Senate floor for a quorum or roll call, on the hard marble floors, became a daily ordeal. In August, a team of physicians from the Lahey Clinic in Boston, visited him on Cape Cod. They described yet another surgery, a complicated procedure to achieve spinal and sacroiliac fusions that, they hoped, would strengthen his lower spine. They explained that without the operation he might lose his ability to walk, but that such a difficult surgery on someone with Addison's Disease posed risks of a fatal infection.

Rose Kennedy said later, "Jack was determined to have the operation. He told his father that even if the risks were fifty-fifty, he would rather be dead than spend the rest of his life hobbling on crutches and paralyzed by pain." Joe tried to dissuade his son from the surgery, reminding him of Franklin Delano Roosevelt's (FDR) extraordinary achievements despite confinement to a wheelchair. After he entered the New York Hospital for special surgery, on October 10, 1954, the team of endocrinologists and surgeons postponed the operation three times in order to do an "extended metabolic work-up prior to, during, and after surgery."

After presurgical evaluations at the Lahey Clinic in Boston, and Bethesda Naval Hospital for special surgery on October 10, he had a three-hour surgery on October 21, 1954.

He was operated on by Dr. Philip D. Wilson. Dr. Ephraim Shorr, his endocrinologist, supervised his hormonal care during and after surgery. The surgery consisted of a double disc fusion wherein bone was grafted, and a metal plate was inserted. JFK described the operation to close friends as "the one that kills you or cures you."

After the surgery, it initially appeared to be uneventful surgery. For three days he was without severe pain or any apparent complication. On the fourth postoperative day, however, he developed a severe infection which did not respond well to antibiotics. JFK lapsed into an unconscious state and was considered critical. The family rushed to the hospital where he was given last rites of the Catholic Church for the second time. JFK proved extraordinarily tough, rallied, and recovered. The surgery had been a big gamble, and his convalescence was prolonged. After the crisis, he remained in the hospital for another two months. He was released from the hospital on December 21, 1954, and continued a meager recovery at the Kennedy Palm Beach home. He spent his Christmas there in great pain, in part, because a complication of the surgery was brewing.

He developed a "staphylococcal infection" at the surgical site which was described by Ted Sorensen, a longtime friend and advisor, as an "*open, gaping very sickly-looking hole*." Lem Billings, JFK's close confidant and friend who visited him during this time stated "*the area where they cut into his back never healed. It was oozing blood and pus all the time. It must have been painful beyond belief...It was an open wound that seemed to be infected all the time. And now and then a piece of bone would come out of the wound. His pain was excruciating.*"

When it became apparent that the open draining wound was infected and not healing, JFK returned to the hospital for a third, less than major, surgery on his back on February 10, 1955. The metal implant was removed, and the infection was treated with antibiotics and debridement.

After three surgeries JFK was essentially in worse shape than before his first surgery in 1944. He continuously required his crutches. He couldn't walk downstairs without assistance. He could barely put weight on his left leg. Fortunately, Dr. Ephraim Shorr took him to see Dr. Janet Travell on May 25, 1955. She was regarded by many of her peers to be the world's top pain and rehabilitation specialist. In 1955 she was probably the only doctor who could save him. She simply knew what to do. It was JFK's lucky day as explained in the next chapter.

Unfortunately, the failed surgery had one more unexpected complication. "Out of the blue." in September 1957 a painful point of redness appeared in the midline operative site of the lumbar spine fusion. It was a superficial lumbar abscess due to a smoldering post-surgical infection. To deal with it, JFK required hospitalization and minor surgery on September 13,

1957. Dr. Preston Wade, a general surgeon, opened the abscess down to the spinal processes of L-4 and L-5 and drained the site. Cultures grew the bacteria, staphylococcus aureus. He was given antibiotics and the abscess healed. This was JFK's last and final surgical procedure.

In summary, JFK underwent two major surgical attempts to cure his back pain The first was in 1944 and the second was ten years later in 1954. He required two minor surgeries after his second major surgery to deal with surgical complications. No surgery decreased his pain. His doctors were mystified over why the surgeries failed and why JFK worsened rather than improved. After the second major surgery in 1954, JFK's endocrinologist, Dr. Ephraim Shorr, knew that death was eminent unless JFK found some relief. He sought out Dr. Janet Travell.

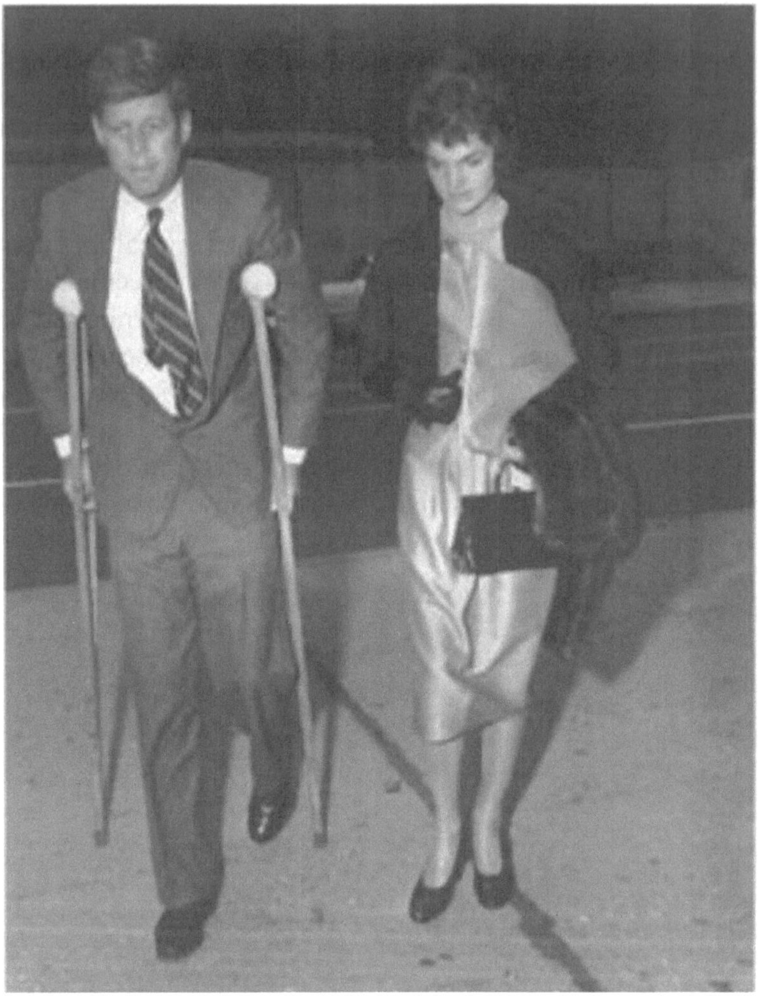

JFK with wife Jackie enter the hospital for his second major spine surgery 1954.

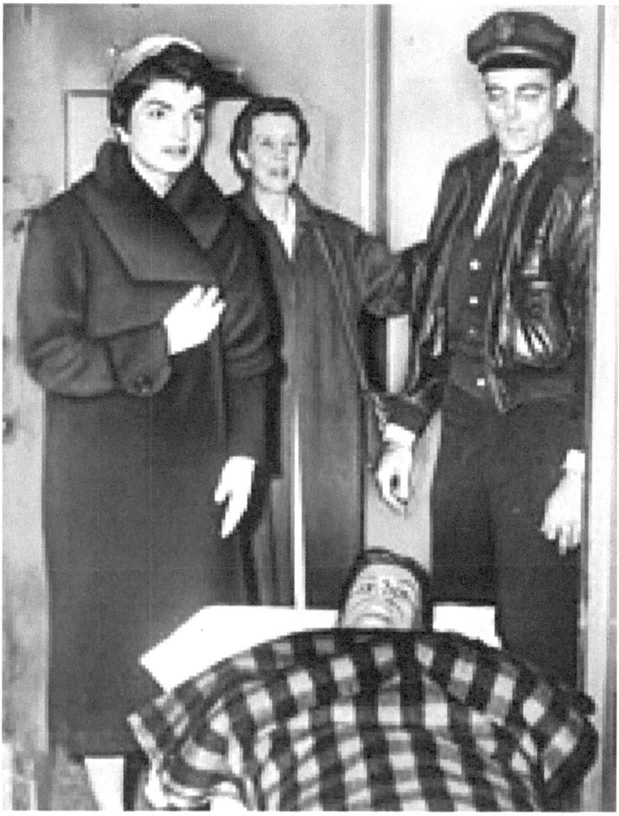

Kennedy and Jackie leaving the hospital following his spinal surgery, December 1954. The surgery did not relieve pain. It was complicated by infection and the implanted metal plate had to be removed.

11. Dr. Janet Travell to The Rescue: 1955–1963 (Ages 37-46)

The Last Stand Works

The Spring of 1955 was the lowest point for JFK in his strange medical saga. Two major spine surgeries had left him with more, rather than less, pain and impairment. He had been given last rites but survived on two occasions. He could hardly turn his body without excruciating pain, and he had to use his crutches to walk. His pain had progressed from being intermittent and controllable to a state of constancy which can erode one's very powers to think and function.[13] He was considering resigning from the Senate. He was simply "down for the count" and "gravesite ready."

Fortunately, his endocrinologist, Ephraim Shorr, MD, was well acquainted with Janet Travell, MD, who, along with her physician father, had been studying back pain and muscle disorders for many years.[36,37] At the time, Dr. Travell was considered by many to be the best pain and rehabilitation specialist in the world.

Dr. Shorr arranged for JFK to meet Dr. Travell at her office in New York City on May 26, 1955. The gods were with JFK that day. On first meeting JFK, Dr. Travell describes his plight in her autobiography.

"Senator Kennedy seemed tired and discouraged. He listened intently but he answered my questions briefly, almost reluctantly, as if he were retelling a boring story. He looked thin; his weight of about 155 pounds did not adequately cover his generous frame and stature of six feet. In spite of his Florida suntan, I thought he appeared pale and anemic, and that indeed proved to be the case. He moved guardedly. He turned his body in one piece when he wanted to face me or Dr. Shorr, Eph and I sat on opposite sides of a wide desk, while his chair was placed at one end. Not only the motion of his back, but also the rotation of his neck was restricted. When I examined him, the reality of his ordeal was brought home to me by the callus under each armpit toward the shoulder blade where the skin had borne his weight on crutches for so long."

Initially when first meeting Dr. Travell, JFK wasn't very impressed. He had gone to scores of doctors who wanted to perform another surgery, nerve block, or prescribe some worthless non-pain-relieving medication. Dr. Travell laments his discouragement.

"He asked a few questions, always to the point. How long would the improvement in the motion of his knee last? He was understandably skeptical. He was not prepared to accept readily one more doctor and another kind of treatment. Seven months earlier he had undergone a lumbar spine fusion, after which a plate had to be removed in a second operation. His crutches had been a familiar sight in the Senate during the summer of a year ago and now he was still obliged to use them."

Dr. Travell wasn't dismayed by JFK's skepticism. After all,

he had come to see Dr. Travell because of what she called his "stubborn hope for better health and respite from pain." After consultation with Dr. Shorr, Dr. Travell felt JFK should immediately enter the hospital to begin medical treatment. Unlike today, in 1955 it was routine to admit a patient to an in-patient setting to initiate aggressive and comprehensive treatment. She started JFK on a broad-based medication, rehabilitation, and exercise program that clearly saved his life, gave him hope, and provided the pain relief he needed to serve as a senator and later become President of the United States.

Dr. Travell's treatments gave JFK not only some relief but hope for a better life. Consequently, Dr. Travell became JFK's primary treating physician between 1955 until his assassination in 1963. Although other physicians participated with certain aspects of his care, she was, however, the backbone of his very survival. Her medical treatment that pulled JFK out of the depths of suffering and likely a death is summarized here.

While in the hospital, in 1955, Dr. Travell began JFK on a potent pain treatment regimen. It included analgesics, physical measures, hormone replacement, sleep induction, and attempts to reduce inflammation. Medical records kept by Dr. Travell over the course of her 8-year treatment reveal that JFK was prescribed the following medications: codeine, meperidine, methadone, methylphenidate, meprobamate, barbiturates, liothyronine, gamma globulin, cortisone, testosterone, and procaine injections. The immediate use of methadone (Dolophine®) and meperidine (Demerol®) were what he needed to function and have a life. Precise dosages, titration schedules, and timing of all JFK's medications are not completely known.

On the day JFK was hospitalized, Dr. Travell took an old-style North Carolina porch rocker to his hospital room much to the amazement of the floor nurses. She colorfully described the incident.

"I parked my car at the delivery entrance to the hospital and

transported the rocking chair up in the freight elevator. The nurses thought it funny to see the chair coming down the hall with the loose rockers, a leather cushion, a sloped footstool, and my medical bag on top, all stacked on the chair seat."

From that time on, Dr. Travell made sure that hardly a day went by without JFK doing a little rocking. The precise therapeutic benefit of "rocking" is believed to enhance lymph and spinal fluid flow and eliminate stasis of biologic waste.[31]

She also highly encouraged him to swim. In late 1955, at the Kennedy home in Palm Beach, she told JFK he was now strong enough to swim in the ocean. Dr. Travell believed that salt water and the lift and fall of ocean swells were a "rocking horse sea." She actually accompanied JFK on his first ocean swim after his surgery. As President, he swam in the White House pool almost daily.

Within about three months after starting Dr. Travell's treatment program, JFK's pain was immensely better. He was back to work as a senator from Massachusetts and planning his run for the presidency. So grateful was JFK and his wife that they invited Dr. Travell to visit with them at their Palm Beach home late in 1955. To emphasize the effectiveness of her treatment she stated in her autobiography: *"I had no idea that before the year (1955) was out I would sit at the table in Palm Beach, where he wrote "Profiles in Courage," in the company of a revitalized John F. Kennedy."*

Several hospitalizations were necessary between 1955 and 1960 to stabilize JFK to the point he could run for the presidency. Eventually his pain was adequately controlled, and he was strong enough to take dozens of campaign trips. What's more, he served 1,000 days as President and only missed one day of work. Any physician today would be proud of this result in such a tragic case.

Dr. Travell recognized that JFK was in severe pain at their very first meeting. From JFK's perspective, he either had to get some pain relief or life wasn't worth living. Dr. Travell knew this, so she immediately hospitalized him to begin pain control. The best pain specialists know that suicide is common in patients who can't obtain pain relief, so she probably was afraid he might end his life if he wasn't observed. Dr. Travell immediately started him on the potent opioid drugs, methadone and meperidine. In recent years, opioids have been highly shunned and condemned, but in the 1950's they were well-accepted in severe pain cases such as JFK. For example, the 1956 "Merck Manual," the desk physician manual, stated relative to pain treatment: *"More severe pain requires the oral or subcutaneous use of codeine, meperidine, methadone, dihydromorphine, metapon, or morphine. The effectiveness of these analgesics often may be enhanced by judicious use of antispasmatics or mild sedatives."*[24]

In addition, the 1955 *Physicians' Desk Reference* categorized pain analgesics for use in cancer, labor, muscular, neuralgic, postoperative, and postpartum conditions.[33] JFK's condition fell under muscular, neuralgic, and postoperative. Dr. Travell's initial opioids included methadonc (Dolophine®), and meperidine (Demerol®). In summary, Dr. Travell's opioid medications were not only standard for the day but stabilized JFK and gave him the will to live and carry on his political career. Robert Kennedy later and rightfully stated that JFK would not have been President if it weren't for Dr. Travell.

In the hands of an experienced physician like Dr. Travell, methadone, meperidine, and codeine can be excellent, long-term pain treatments. JFK was a clear benefactor. Methadone is a long-acting opioid that provides great stability to a pain patient whose pain is constant, intractable, and interferes with daily living.[14] It provides potent pain suppression in a person such as JFK who has a demanding schedule. Meperidine is an excellent fast-acting, short-duration opioid that can extinguish pain flares or what is sometimes called "breakthrough" pain. Dr. Travell's pain treatment obviously gave JFK enough pain relief to campaign and later serve as President of the United States.

Although Dr. Travell wisely first tackled JFK's debilitating and demoralizing pain with an opioid regimen and a rocking chair, she set out in 1955 to build an all-encompassing therapeutic program. JFK suffered from both insomnia and muscle spasms which are typical in persons with severe, constant pain. She prescribed a barbiturate (Tuinal®) to get some sleep. Dr. Travell well-recognized that JFK had to have some decent sleep to carry out his political duties.

Many severe pain patients can't get adequate relief without the use of a stimulant. In 1896 physicians at the Brompton Hospital in London recognized that substantive pain control usually required the simultaneous administration of an opioid and a stimulant. JFK was prescribed methylphenidate (Ritalin®), which is still used today in palliative pain patients. It is now widely recognized that stimulants such as an amphetamine derivative, provide considerable pain relief in intractable pain patients.[33] Their mechanism of action is to enhance the neurotransmitters, dopamine and noradrenaline.

Dr. Travell believed JFK had a peripheral neuritis caused by vitamin B deficiencies when she first examined him in 1955. Her basis was loss of vibratory sensation in his legs. She prescribed B and C vitamins including B_{12}. She gave him a diagnosis of pernicious anemia which is highly associated with Addison's disease.[1] Dr. Travell also believed JFK had a thyroid deficiency. Typical symptoms are lethargy, ankle swelling, depression, and dry skin. She prescribed liothyronine, a thyroid derivative, beginning in 1955.

At the time JFK came under Dr. Travell's care, he was taking cortisone and prednisone for his Addison's Disease. She and Dr. Shorr, and later Dr. Eugene Cohen, continued to prescribe these hormones until his death in 1963.

Besides pain relief, Dr. Travell was an expert at physical rehabilitation measures.[36] She had a keen interest in how shoes, chairs, and braces put stress on back muscles. She observed that JFK was born with a left leg about an inch shorter than his right. Although the deformity was noticed at birth but was never an issue with any of his physicians prior to Dr. Travell. She made him a heel lift to keep him balanced. She designed special chairs with a writing table attached so he could sit and write without back strain. JFK used a variety of back braces and corsets, which Dr. Travell designed. She started procaine injections, heat, and ultrasound when his back pain flared.

The gastrointestinal symptoms, including nausea, bloating, pain, and diarrhea, that began in JFK's childhood continued to periodically flare. Dr. Travell took over care for this ailment and prescribed atropine and diphenoxylate. She was an expert in the use of procaine injections for pain that is anatomically located in one area.[36] She would inject his back up to six times a day if he was in a severe pain flare. In the 1950's procaine injections became quite popular. JFK initially felt the procaine injections were a godsend. Dr. Travell started the injections in 1955 just after his surgeries. The injections would give JFK pain relief for several hours which allowed him to run for President. At one point JFK called Dr. Travell a genius because of the shots. The 1955 *Physicians' Desk Reference* said this about procaine injections.

"Procaine hydrochloride, one of the oldest drugs in current use, continues to be the local anesthetic of choice for many infiltration and other anesthetic procedures. Recently it has also been used with a high degree of success as an analgesic and therapeutic agent. Procaine has proved effective in relieving arthritic symptoms, controlling postoperative pain, easing edema, and pain of trauma."

At some point, Dr. Travell and Drs. Shorr and Cohen, her consulting endocrinologists, started JFK on testosterone derivatives. It is unknown whether JFK's original complaint was impotence, loss of libido, or failure to gain weight. There were no laboratory tests for testosterone blood levels during JFK's life, so his physicians, Dr. Travell and Cohen, started him on testosterone derivatives based on symptoms. His first derivative was oral methyltestosterone. Others were later attempted. JFK fathered four children while under Dr. Travell's care, so there is little evidence that his sexual abilities were greatly impaired.

Another problem that constantly befell JFK was chronic urinary-prostate discharge. This condition was treated with gamma globulin and periodic antibiotics. The precise cause of the discharge was never pinned down.

Dr. Travell and her fellow physicians had to treat JFK on symptoms. The "diagnostic age" of medicine with a plethora of blood, electronic, urine, and magnetic resonance imaging (MRI) tests were not yet invented. Not until the 21st century could medical experts even determine that JFK had a genetic, autoimmune polyglandular syndrome and the horrible complication of adhesive arachnoiditis because laboratory tests were simply not yet available. Autoimmunity was not recognized in JFK's lifetime. It is simply defined as "an intrinsic body mechanism that automatically rusts and impairs some tissue". The concept of autoimmunity did not gain wide acceptance until the 1970's and 80's.[20,21]

The 1962 edition of Dorland's Medical Dictionary does not even list autoimmune disease.[9] The 1965 edition of Current Therapy only refers to "autoimmune reactions."[15] Slowly but surely the medical profession began to accept the fact that the body may actually turn on itself. In contrast to the 1962 edition, Dorland's Medical Dictionary in 1981 defined autoimmunity as "a condition characterized by a specific humoral or cell-mediated immune response against the constituents of the body's own tissues."[10] By 1989, Taber's Medical dictionary succinctly defined autoimmune disease as we view it today: "Disease in which the body produces (a) disordered immunological response against itself."[31] Today it is known that autoimmunity and severe pain go hand-in-hand.[35]

Dr. Travell's treatment program was necessarily complex. She literally rescued JFK as he was near death due to his medical conditions as well as possibly considering suicide. Attached is a Summary Table of her overall medical program. Dr. Lee Mandell, a Naval endocrinologist, reviewed Dr. Travell's records in 2008 and published a single day's detailed account of her complex medical treatment on October 12, 1961.

"He was taking ascorbic acid (vitamin C), 500 mg twice daily; hydrocortisone, 10 mg daily; prednisone, 2.5 mg twice daily; methyltestosterone, 10 mg/d; liothyronine sodium, 25 ug twice daily; fludrocortisone, 0,1 mg/d; and diphenoxylate hydrochloride and atropine sulfate, 2 tablets as needed."

<u>Table of Abbreviations</u>

mg = milligrams
mg/d = milligrams per day
ug = micrograms

Interestingly, the three cortisone derivatives taken in a single day, cortisone, prednisone, and fludrocortisone represent total hormone replacement for non-functional adrenal glands (ie Addison's). Indeed, his autopsy in 1963, about two years later, showed essentially total atrophy of both adrenals.

After JFK was inaugurated as President in January 1961, the stress of the job caused more back pain. Unfortunately, the procaine injections were starting to lose their power and effectiveness. In June of 1961, JFK was in Ottawa for a ceremonial tree planting when he bent over to shovel a small amount of dirt, he threw out his back. His pain flared and he even had to resort to his crutches. Drs. George Burkley and Eugene Cohen, the other White House physicians, wanted to call in a physical therapist and stop procaine injections. Dr. Travell initially rejected this opinion, because physical therapy is always a "hit and miss" proposition when it comes to pain relief. She finally and reluctantly called in Dr. Hans Kraus, a noted orthopedic surgeon and physical therapist, who was recommended by the White House endocrinologist, Dr. Cohen. This proved to be a good move as Dr. Kraus was able to bring another medical dimension to JFK's medical program. Details are in a later chapter.

In summary, the importance of Dr. Travell's treatment program can't be overemphasized. It was complex and very advanced. She clearly brought JFK out of despair and agony. She restored him to a healthy enough state to campaign and serve as President. Robert Kennedy said it best, "If it had not been for her, JFK would not have been President." It is noted here that Dr. Travell had a famed career after the death of JFK. She continued to study back injections and find safer alternatives to procaine. She became an icon among physicians and was sometimes called the "Mother of Trigger Points." She lectured widely and taught the next generation of physicians, including the author of this book, the value of trigger point injections. Her book published in 1984 called "Myofascial Pain and Dysfunctions: The Trigger Point Manuel" continues to this day to be a seminal manual for physicians who do pain management and trigger point injections.

SUMMARY OF DR. TRAVELL'S TREATMENT PROGRAM	
PHYSICAL EXERCISES	Rocking chair, Swimming, Muscle stretching/strengthening
MEDICATIONS	
Opioids	Methadone (Dolophine®), Meperidine (Demerol®), Codeine
Bedtime sedative/sleeping aid	Barbiturates (Tuinal®)
Muscle relaxants/anxiety	Meprobamate (Miltown®), chlordiazepoxide (Librium®)
Topical/local anesthesia	Procaine injections
Stimulant	Methylphenidate (Ritalin®)
Hormones	Cortisone, Desoxycorticosterone Acetate, implants, Prednisone, Methyltestosterone, Liothyronine
GASTROINTESTINAL SYMPTOMS	Atropine, dyphenoxylate
INFECTION CONTROL	Gamma globulin
VITAMINS	B_{12}, B complex, C
REHABILITATION MEASURES	Heel lift, back brace and corset, special chairs

The above program was initiated in 1955 and was progressively enhanced until JFK's death in 1963. All drugs and measures may not be shown here.

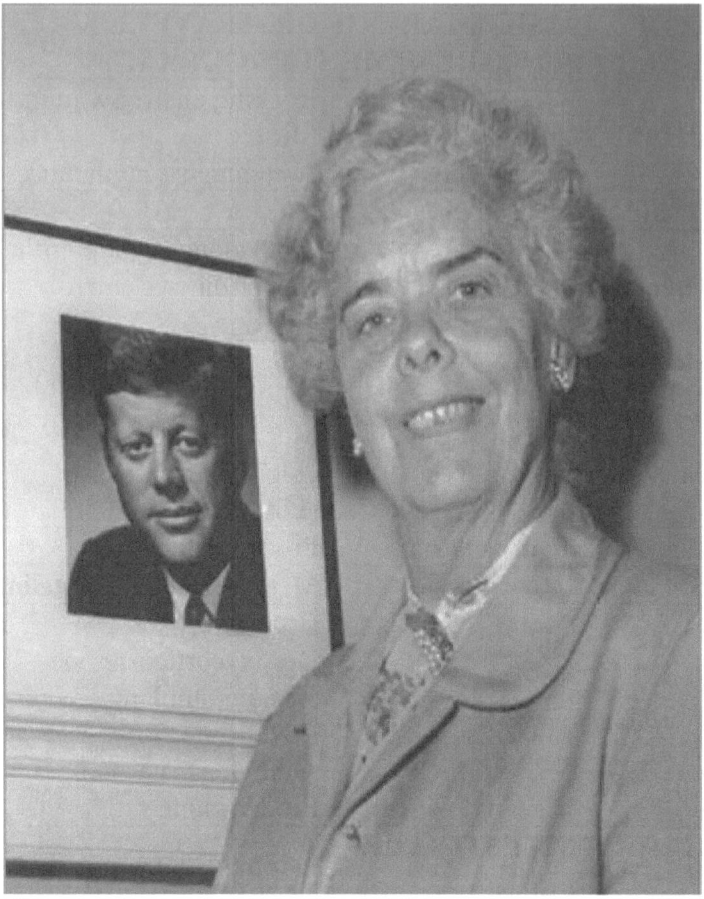

Dr. Janet Travell began effective pain treatment after his second, failed major spine surgery.
In 1955. She cared for JFK until his death in 1963.

12. Dr. Max Jacobson: Performance Enhancement 1960-1963 (Ages 42-46)

Saving the Presidential Campaign

JFK had seen scores of physicians in his lifetime, but he only invited two physicians to his Presidential inauguration. His primary physician and the one who pulled him from the abyss of near death, Dr. Travell, was there. A second physician, Dr. Max Jacobson, was in attendance. He provided JFK with a medical cocktail that gave him energy and stamina to campaign for the Presidency.

Little is known about Dr. Jacobson because his story, to this day, is one that remains somewhat mysterious, shocking, and controversial. During his lifetime two common names were applied to him to describe his treatments – "Dr. Feelgood" or "Miracle Max". JFK believed that Dr. Jacobson's treatments greatly benefitted him and made it possible for him to function as the President.

Dr. Jacobson's notoriety stems from his development and use of an injectable concoction or cocktail that would come to be called a "performance enhancing drug or cocktail." His cocktail contained methamphetamine, human chorionic gonadotropin (HCG), calcium, and niacin, and probably some other vitamins, hormones, and corticosteroids. Precise dosages and ingredients are not known. HCG was extracted from horse urine or from a placenta that he kept in his personal laboratory. Dr. Jacobson never released his formulas as he considered them to be proprietary. Also, he likely varied them from patient-to-patient as he made his own solutions and marketed them in vials. Published reports say he kept placenta and perhaps other biologic materials in his laboratory refrigerator, from which to make his cocktails.

In 2013, Richard Lertzman and William Birnes wrote an in-depth book entitled "Dr. Feelgood." These authors painstakingly unearthed much of the history and many of Dr. Jacobson's secrets. They understandably allege that his "performance enhancing cocktail" was used by so many famous leaders that Dr. Jacobson singlehandedly may have influenced world events.

Dr. Jacobson's connection to the Kennedys began in 1960 when JFK was campaigning for the Presidency. At this time, he had been under Dr. Travell's care for about four years. His overall health was holding up well enough to campaign for the Presidency with little progression of his basic conditions although he had constant pain and carried a recurrent urinary tract infection. The campaign, however, was stressful to his ravaged spine. His adrenal glands just couldn't take the stress of the campaign. He became exhausted and fearful that he couldn't compete with his opponent, Richard Nixon, whom he was to debate in the first nationally televised, Presidential debate. JFK's close friend, Chuck Spalding, placed a confidential phone call to Dr. Jacobson and requested a private consultation on behalf of an unidentified friend. Mr. Spalding communicated that this "friend" was in a tight situation and needed Dr.

Jacobson's assistance. Prior to this phone call JFK had complained to Mr. Spalding about a progressive loss of stamina and fatigue brought on by his grueling campaign. Mr. Spalding himself was a patient of Dr. Jacobson's and took pains to ensure that JFK could be seen by him with utmost secrecy.

Dr. Jacobson's office was on East 72nd Street in New York. He was quite open with his patients, media, or anyone who asked if his specialty was treating stress. His office was described by "Lertzman-Birnes" as a celebrity waiting room with a research lab. The lab was there to allow Dr. Jacobson to extract compounds from tissues such as placenta and mix his cocktails to be distributed in vials for injection or sublingual (under-the-tongue) drops.

JFK first visited Dr. Jacobson in the summer of 1960 just a few weeks before the famous Nixon-Kennedy debate. He complained to Dr. Jacobson about the demands of the campaign. It was draining him. He was fatigued, muscles were weak, and his weakness was interfering with his concentration and his speech. Also, he was getting laryngitis due to incessant speaking on the campaign trail.

Dr. Jacobson took a short medical history. JFK told the doctor about his chronic back pain and Addison's disease and how they resulted in extreme weakness, fluctuating blood pressure, chronic nausea, and diarrhea. He needed pain relief medication to be able to walk without crutches. JFK also told Dr. Jacobson about his extensive and effective medical regimen prescribed or supervised by Dr. Travell. This included corticosteroids for Addison's disease, opioids for pain, sleep aids, antibiotics for a chronic urinary tract infection, and thyroid for fatigue.

JFK had no reluctance in accepting Dr. Jacobson's treatment. Besides his friend Chuck Spalding, JFK had likely been in contact with some of the doctor's other famous patients (See the attached Table) who had been treated for their stress. Dr.

Jacobson injected JFK on their first visit. It took effect immediately. JFK had entered the office tired and weak, but suddenly it relieved most of his pain. He was also able to move more easily, and felt stronger, focused, and alert. JFK suddenly felt like a new person with some relief and hope. He was immediately sold on Dr. Jacobson's cocktail like many other famous people before him. Most important, he now knew he could take the stress of a Presidential campaign.

Dr. Jacobson sent JFK home with a dropper bottle of his medical concoction for JFK to periodically use by placing drops under his tongue.

JFK visited Dr. Jacobson on the evening of September 26, 1960, just a couple of hours before his first debate with Richard Nixon. His voice had been reduced to barely a whisper, and he complained of fatigue and lethargy. Dr. Jacobson injected his cocktail directly into JFK's throat to pump up his larynx (voice box). The injection immediately strengthened his voice and gave him the energy and vigor to engage in debate. About seventy million people, including this author, watched Kennedy beat Nixon. JFK appeared young, alert, healthy, and clearly fit to be the next President.

Unknown to anyone else, JFK had found something, the Dr. Jacobson cocktail, that gave him some relief from his pain and misery and allowed him to perform at his best while in the public eye. He wasn't about to give it up. From that day forward he became a regular patient of Dr. Jacobson. He made sure that Dr. Jacobson was at his inauguration in case he had a severe flare of pain, fatigue, and exhaustion.

After JFK and his wife entered the White House in January 1961 to be the 35th President of the United States. Dr. Jacobson became his other personal physician along with Dr. Travell. While Dr. Travell had an official White House title, Dr. Jacobson did not. He would, however, periodically attend JFK and his wife during the 1000 days they occupied the White

House. In phone conversations between JFK and Dr. Jacobson, JFK was known as "Mrs. Dunn."

During Dr. Jacobson's frequent visits to the White House, he taught JFK how to inject his cocktail into his buttocks. It is unknown as to the frequency that JFK self-administered the injections. It is known that JFK came to rely on the cocktail for stressful situations. He even had Dr. Jacobson as well as Dr. Travell accompany him to Paris in 1961 to help him through his negotiations with Nikita Khrushchev, the Russian Leader. It is reported that he took injections just before meeting him as JFK had come to believe that Dr. Jacobson's medication aided his performance just as musicians or athletes may take a performance enhancing drug(s) just before a performance. For example, Dr. Arnold Mandell published a book entitled "The Nightmare Season" in which he describes the use of amphetamine derivatives by the San Diego Charger football team. Elvis Presley used amphetamine derivatives before some performances.

Human chorionic gonadotropin (HCG), a hormone produced in placental tissues, was part of Dr. Jacobson's cocktail. Today it is considered an "anabolic steroid" and is used in high dosages by athletes and body builders to look and feel better. Its popularity is described in Dr. Robert Kerr's book on the athletic use of anabolic steroids. In lower dosages it is used for pain reduction and weight control purposes. Dr. Jacobson extracted HCG from placental tissues and/or from horse urine kept in his laboratory. HCG is produced in the placenta of pregnant women to help the fetus grow a nervous system and to provide on-going pain relief during pregnancy as the uterus expands.

Based on his actions, JFK considered Drs. Travell and Jacobson to both be equal and critically important to his ability to function and survive. Dr. Travell and the other physicians who attended JFK, however, did not approve of Dr. Jacobson or his treatments. At one point they resented Dr. Jacobson partly because he refused to reveal the ingredients of his cocktail as well as his unorthodox and unprofessional demeanor. He never socialized with the other White House physicians, and he was reputed to look like a "mad scientist" with dirty fingernails and a lab coat stained with chemicals. His back office was unkept and placenta and other tissues were kept in his laboratory refrigerator. At one point Dr. Travell and the other White House physicians admonished JFK to stop Dr. Jacobson's injections. JFK refused by saying, "I don't care if it is horse piss, it works." The reference to urine is likely that horse urine was a usual source of HCG. Interestingly, since Jacobson also used placenta extracts, other hormones besides HCG may have been in his cocktail.

Lertzman and Birnes went to great lengths to understand the allure of Dr. Jacobson's cocktail. They interviewed many people, including famous ones, as to why they patronized Dr. Jacobson. The renowned singer, Eddie Fisher, referred to Dr. Jacobson as "Miracle Max." The diligent researchers published a list of the personalities they could identify as being treated by Dr. Jacobson. That list is attached because it is erroneous to believe that JFK used a treatment that was poorly accepted at the time. Part of the strange medical saga of JFK is that he was in "lockstep" with a lot of famous people that are highly remembered and revered in American society.

Lertzman and Birnes described some of the feelings and allure of Dr. Jacobson's cocktail. Eddie Fisher said the injections felt as if he was being "lit from within." Truman Capote described it as "Instant euphoria, you feel like Superman. You're flying. Ideas come at the speed of light. You go 72 hours straight without so much as a coffee break. You don't need sleep; you don't need nourishment. If it's sex you're after, you go all night." Harvey Mann, a part-time actor and employee of Dr. Jacobson described the effects of the injection as "it gives you the initial flash, the needle actually feels red hot going in, and you get a reaction in your testicles just like an orgasm, your testicles feel hot as hell, your feet rise above the ground, you feel like you're in heat, like you could have multiple orgasms. It's the calcium-niacin combination that gives you that, and it's no wonder those injections hooked all of us."

Lertzman and Birnes described several who got "hooked" or "addicted" in that they shifted from occasional to daily multiple injections. They believed that methamphetamine in the injections was the compelling ingredient that led to the addictive use of Dr. Jacobson's injections. Methamphetamine abuse and addiction are now a well-known tragedy, so their conclusion is likely correct. It is unknown how often JFK used the injections, or if he used them often enough to qualify for a definition of "addiction."

Lertzman and Birnes firmly believed that Dr. Jacobson and his cocktail had influenced some historical events, simply because so many famous and important people used his cocktail. The idea is that the cocktail allowed the rich and famous to make a decision or engage in an activity they would otherwise not have done. Certainly, no one can authoritatively refute this premise.

Dr. Jacobson's medical practice was perfectly legal in the 1950's and 60's. He clearly was successful in creating a concoction that attracted some of Society's top leaders. He never revealed his precise formula, and he may have varied it from patient-to-patient and time-to-time. He considered his drugs and practice to be a rightful, entrepreneurial endeavor. JFK was certainly grateful and gave Dr. Jacobson a tie clip with a PT109 insignia on it.

In 1972, the Federal Controlled Substance Act was passed that banned his doctor's ability to order methamphetamine and make his own formulas. Also, the New York Medical Board had received so many complaints about his medications and operations that his license to practice was rescinded. He died in 1979.

Despite the many controversies regarding Dr. Jacobson, one thing stands out relative to JFK. There is no evidence that his treatments injured, damaged, or impaired JFK. In fact, JFK's overall health steadily improved between the time Dr. Travell took over his care in 1955 and his death eight years later in 1963. There were several doctors involved in his care during this time, so it is difficult to know what worked and what did not. This eight-year period, compared to other periods of his life didn't require hospitalization, surgery, or bed bound days. He reportedly missed only one day of work out of the 1000 days he served as President. Despite Dr. Jacobson's controversies, the evidence suggests his treatments positively contributed to JFK's progressive health improvement during his Presidency.

Max Jacobson Patient List

(Reference: Lertzman RA, Birnes WJ. Dr. Feelgood. Stayhorse Publishing, New York, 213,pp175-177.

Alan Jay Lerner
Allice Ghostley*
Anais Nin
Andy Warhol
Andy Williams*
Anthony Quinn
Arlene Francis
Arnold Saint-Subber
Billy Wilder*
Bob Cummings*
Bob Fosse
Bob Richardson
Burgess Meredith
Burton Lane
Cary Grant
Cecil B. DeMille
Chuck Spalding
Cicely Tyson
Claude Pepper
Doris Shapiro
Dorothy McGuire
Eddie albert
Eddie Fisher*
Edie Sedgewick
Edward G. Robinson
Elizabeth Taylor*
Ellen Hanley
Elvis Presley
Emilio Pucci
Eusebio Morales
Everly Bros.
Felice Orlandi
Franchot Tone
Franco Zifferelle
Frank Sinatra
George Kaufman
Gore Vidal
Greta Stuckles
Gypsy Rose Lee (Rose Havoc)
Harry S. Truman
Hedy Lamarr
Henry and June Miller
Henry Morgan
Hermione Gingold
Howard Cosell
Hugh Martin
Igor Goran
Igor Stravinsky
Ingrid Bergman
Jacqueline Kennedy
Jerry Lewis*
John f. Kennedy
John Hancock (director)
John Murray Anderson
Johnny Mathis
Jose Ferrer
Josh Logan
Judith Exner Campbell
Judy Garland
Katherine Dunham
Kay Thompson
Kurt Braun
Lee Bouvier Radziwill*
Leonard Bernstein
Leontyne Price
Louis Nizer
Mabel Mercer
Margaret Leighton
Marianne Anderson
Marilyn Monroe
Marilyn Marlowe
Mark Shaw
Marlene Dietrich
Martin Gabel
Maya Deren
Maynard Ferguson
Mel Allen

Mickey Mantle
Mike Todd
Milton Blackstone
Nancy Olson
Nelson Rockefeller
Niels Bohr
Otto Preminger
Pat Suzuki*
Patrick O'Neil
Paul Lynde
Paul Robeson
Peter Lawford
Peter Lorre
Phyllis McGuire
Rebekah Harkness
Richard Burton
Richard M. Nixon
Rita Moreno
Robert Goulet
Rod Serling
Roddy McDowell*
Ronny Graham
Rosalind Russell
Roscoe Lee Browne*
Rosemary Clooney
Roy Cohn
Sam "MoMo" Giancanna
Sharon Tate
Shelley Winters
Spiro Agnew
Stash Radziwill
Stavros Niachros
Tennessee Williams
Tom Parker
Tony Curtis*
Tony Franciosa
Truman Capote
Van Cliburn
Vic Damone
Vincent Alo ("Jimmy Blue Eyes")
Winston Churchill
Yul Brynner
Zero Mostel

*Interviewed by the authors

This list, according to the authors of the book "Dr. Feelgood" came from office records kept by Dr. Jacobson.

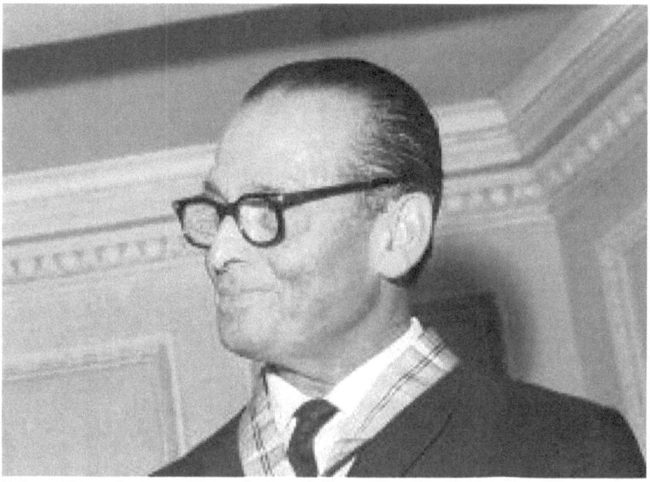

Dr. Max Jacobson developed "cocktails" that relieved stress and fatigue and enhanced JFK's speaking and debate performances. JFK found the "cocktail" aided his health until his death.

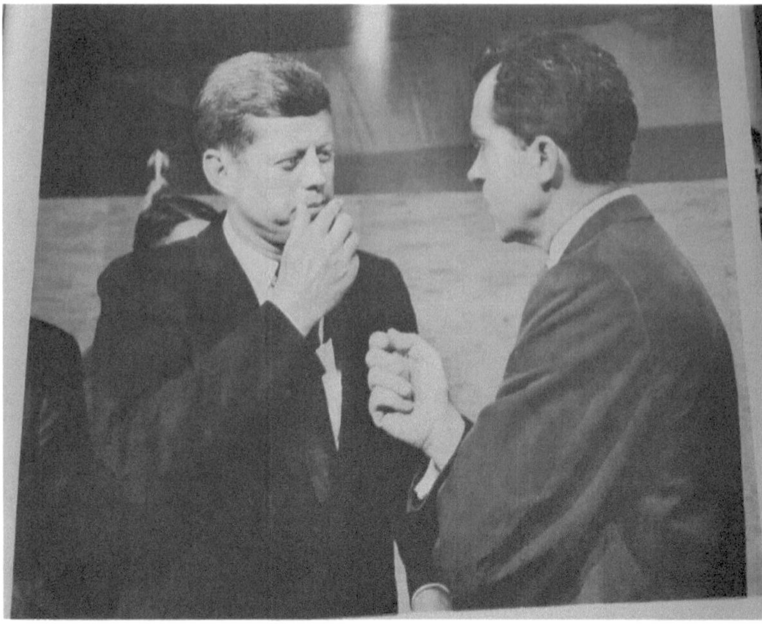

JFK and Richard Nixon converse at a Presidential debate in 1960.

13. White House Care: 1961-1963 (Ages 43-46)

Chaotic But Effective

At 8:00 AM on the day after JFK was sworn in as President, he made his first Presidential appointment. He took the unusual step of awarding Dr. Travell with two positions on his White House medical team: (1) Chief White House Physician and (2) the White House Back Doctor. Dr. Travell was the first woman ever appointed to a White House medical team.

Some Washington insiders were shocked. Dr. Travell was an unusual choice for the top medical role both because she was practicing as a specialist instead of a generalist in internal medicine and a civilian instead of a military doctor. The Washington Post noted, "The appointment ruffled a few feathers among members of the Washington establishment, especially in the military, which had regularly staffed the White House position since the early 1920's.

Although it was natural for JFK to appoint the physician who had saved his life and helped him in his campaign, he was obviously not acquainted with all the duties of the Chief White House Physician. As much as anything it is an administrative position in charge of a sizeable medical complex. Also, the Chief White House Physician needs some rank and experience to "get things done" in the tangled bureaucracy of the Federal Government. It was generally assumed that the White House physician's job would go to Dr. George Burkley who was a Naval Captain but promoted to Rear Admiral in August 1961. He was a holdover from the Eisenhower administration, and he was a cardiologist-internist. Despite his superb qualifications for the job he became Dr. Travell's assistant.

Besides Drs. Travell and Burkley, JFK brought on his endocrinologist, Dr. Eugene Cohen. A fourth doctor was unofficially on JFK's medical team, Dr. Max Jacobson who had given JFK his performance enhancing cocktail that helped him defeat Richard Nixon in debate. Over the 1000 days in the White House, there was considerable contempt and disagreements regarding JFK's treatments among the physicians. Drs. Travell, Burkley, and Cohen did agree on one thing. They neither personally cared for Dr. Max Jacobson, nor the fact that he would periodically enter the White House and give JFK his cocktail. At one confrontation JFK let everyone know he was sticking with Dr. Jacobson and said, "I don't care if it is horse piss, it works." This was a reference to the fact that human chorionic gonadotropin (HCG) and perhaps other hormones were, in these years, extracted from horse urine.

Some chaos and contempt between Drs. Travell, Burkley, and Cohen broke out within six months after JFK took office. Shortly after JFK took office his back pain began to unmercifully relapse perhaps because of the strain of the presidency. It really "whacked out" in June 1961 when he bent over to shovel a small amount of dirt in a tree planting ceremony in Ottawa, Canada. Dr. Travell would need to inject his back sometimes two or three times a day to give him some relief. By mid-year 1961, Dr. Burkley noted that the procaine injections as well as his back brace weren't helping like they once did. Dr. Burkley along with endocrinologist, Dr. Cohen, demanded that Dr. Travell bring in a consultant to attempt physical therapy on JFK's back. She initially refused, but Dr. Burkley with the support of Dr. Cohen persuaded her to accept the fact that they needed a new approach to JFK's back care. The procaine injections had lost their effectiveness, and the President's functional abilities were starting to fail. Dr. Travell finally relented, and in late 1961 brought on Dr. Hans Kraus, an orthopedic surgeon who specialized in back rehabilitation. The next chapter provides details of Dr. Kraus' treatments.

It is not precisely clear when the changes occurred, but JFK had Drs. Burkley and Travell switch jobs. Dr. Burkley was put in charge and Dr. Travell made his assistant. Dr. Kraus was made head back doctor. Dr. Burkley was publicly made JFK's personal physician in June 1963. Over time it became clear to JFK and the civilian doctors why a high-ranking military doctor needed to be in charge. Civilian doctors simply aren't prepared for the boiler-room politics of the White House. At that time Dr. James M. Young, a thirty-three-year-old Naval Captain, was appointed White House Physician. Dr. Travell stayed on, however, as her complex and effective medical and pain program had to continue on. The other doctors, particularly Dr. Burkley, recognized her skills and good results generated by her and the other physicians, even Dr. Jacobson.

As JFK's personal physician, Dr. Burkley accompanied him to Dallas and was in the car behind JFK during the ill-fated motorcade. When JFK was shot Dr. Burkley showed why he was also an Admiral. He almost singlehandedly took charge immediately after JFK was shot. He ignored the chaos and got his contingency to take the President and Jackie to Parkland Hospital. After he was declared dead, he immediately had JFK placed in a brass casket and flown to Washington, DC. Dr. Burkley traveled with Jackie Kennedy who gave permission for an autopsy and requested it be done at the Bethesda Naval

Hospital rather than the Armed Forces Institute of Pathology. It is reported that Jackie Kennedy wanted the autopsy done at the Naval hospital because her husband was a Navy man. Dr. Burkley, with his Admiral rank commanded the pathologists who did the autopsy to have their report on his desk within twenty-four hours. They complied.

Despite some contempt, disagreements, and shifting of titles between the five physicians who attended JFK in the White House in his 1000-day tenure, they got the job done. The evidence for this is that JFK's health continued to progressively improve since Dr. Travell became his main doctor in 1955. Her medical program was complex and intense. It required multiple hormonal replacements, potent pain relief medications, and the muscle and strength building that Dr. Kraus brought in when it appeared that JFK could slip back into severe pain, crutches, and despair. In summary, JFK's White House care may have been chaotic and contentious, but it worked. He was in the best health ever when he was assassinated. In the 1000 days he served as President, he only missed one day of work, didn't require a hospitalization, and above all, didn't need another issuance of "last rites." An unsung and unappreciated hero in the medical chaos of JFK's administration was Admiral (Dr.) George Burkley. JFK had recruited the best civilian doctors available to treat his rare conditions, but it took a high-ranking, medical officer to keep them in line.

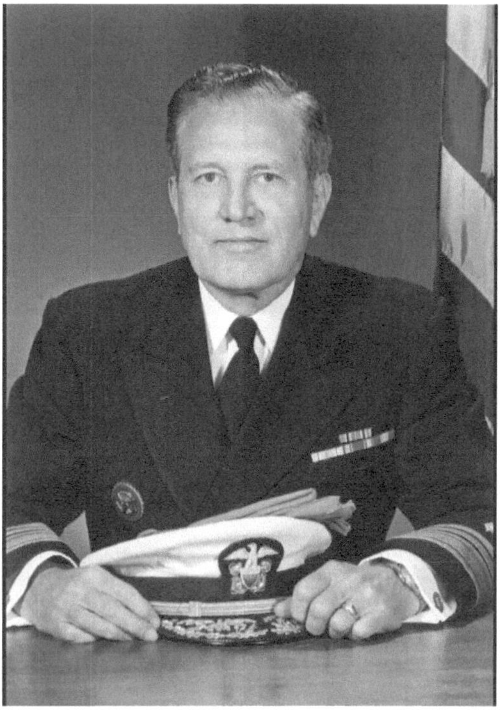

Dr. (US Naval Admiral) George Burkley, served on JFK's medical team during his White House years and coordinated his post-assassination autopsy. He also cared for Presidents Eisenhower and Johnson.

14. Dr. Hans Kraus Builds Strength 1961–1963 (Ages 44-46)

Saving the Presidency

The White House physicians faced a medical dilemma in mid-1961 after JFK developed back spasms and disabling pain after attending a tree planting ceremony in Ottawa, Canada. He bent over to shovel a small amount of dirt and he "threw out his back," which meant he either herniated a disc, tore some nerves that enter or exit the spinal cord, or ripped some muscles in the lower back. The precise diagnosis of a "thrown back" can't always be determined even in today's high tech medical world. Regardless, it was clear that JFK was in serious trouble relative to carrying out his Presidential duties. He had constant pain, walked stiffly, rose from a chair with difficulty, resorted to his crutches, and spent a lot of time in the heated White House pool. To his physicians the issue was that JFK's treatments of the past no longer worked well. Dr. Travell found that even a half dozen procaine injections a day didn't do much. Ultrasound, heat, and even opioid medications did little or nothing to relieve his pain.

No one considered surgery as his two major spine surgeries were abominable failures. In short, as a desperate gambler might say, "I'm out of aces".

The three White House physicians, Drs. Travell, Burkley, and Cohen were frightened and frustrated over the inability to find something that would permit JFK to keep functioning as a President should. They disagreed on what to do and some arguments and dissention broke out between them. Dr. Cohen, the endocrinologist, had previously worked with a physical medicine specialist named Dr. Hans Kraus in New York City where he had been in private practice before joining the White House medical team. He wanted to bring in Dr. Kraus who had a reputation in some medical circles as a physical therapy "whiz kid" when it came to treating bad backs. At first Dr. Travell, the head physician, didn't go for this idea. After a while, however, Drs. Burkley and Cohen prevailed upon her to bring him on board. Even though Dr. Burkley was not officially the White House head physician, as a high-ranking Naval officer and knowledgeable doctor, he was a persuasive figure who could get things done. He persuaded Dr. Travell to try something new. It was hard for Dr. Travell to accept the fact that her innovative procaine injections just didn't work very well anymore. Undoubtedly, the nerves in the back muscles of JFK had become tolerant and resistant to procaine over the years. Drs. Burkley and Cohen thought that the dozens of procaine injections may actually have damaged his back. As this author can attest, it's a sad, personal day for a physician to realize and admit that his/her favorite treatment may "run out of steam" and you need a consultation. Dr. Travell, much to her credit and leadership, finally agreed to bring in Dr. Kraus. She and other physicians agreed to let him do "his thing" while they continued their medical and endocrine therapies. JFK insisted that Dr. Jacobson's performance enhancing cocktail was essential, so he continued his periodic visits during the same time Dr. Kraus treated JFK's back.

On October 14, 1961, Dr. Travell called Dr. Kraus, and the

next day he flew to Washington and examined JFK. Dr. Travell met Dr. Kraus at the airport, and she set up a temporary shop for him in her office. Dr. Kraus started a medical record which he kept in his New York office away from the White House. His top line read "K" and he was 44 years old, six feet tall, and weighed 179 pounds. Dr. Kraus diligently examined JFK's back muscles for weakness, trigger points, and distortion. He put JFK through some strength and limb extension tests and watched how he moved and walked. Interestingly, he wasn't interested in reviewing Dr. Travell's records or viewing x-rays. Dr. Kraus was old-fashioned. He put his faith in his physical exam. It told him a lot about JFK's health and relapse. He found JFK to have such a weak back and stomach muscles that he couldn't do a single sit up and his leg muscles felt "as taut as piano wires." When Dr. Kraus asked him to bend forward and touch his toes, he couldn't even reach his knees.

Dr. Kraus was an unusual physician. He was a short man about five-foot six and very muscular. He was European born and trained at the Vienna University Hospital. Prior to treating JFK, he treated many celebrities. Mike Wallace of TV fame once said, "anyone who was anyone went to Kraus." The amazing attribute of Dr. Kraus was that he loved physical activity and he himself was an expert rock climber. To Dr. Kraus good medical treatment was principally physical and endurance training

After Dr. Kraus did his old-fashioned physical exam, he told JFK "You will be a cripple soon if you don't start exercising five days a week. And you need to start now."

Dr. Kraus met with the White House physicians and gave them an ultimatum. He wanted absolute control with no interference from the other White House doctors. Otherwise, he would not work with JFK. Dr. Kraus had a commanding demeanor, so they didn't doubt his claim and they all gave him full authority. They kept their word. They had a deteriorating President on their hands, and they had no alternative medical measures to offer as their medical bags were pretty light at this time.

At the time Dr. Kraus came on board, Dr. Burkley switched roles with Dr. Travell as the Chief White House Physician although this move wasn't publicized. Drs. Travell, Cohen, and Jacobson continued JFK's complex medical program.

After Dr. Kraus accepted the assignment to treat JFK, Dr. Burkley set up a small area next to the swimming pool where Dr. Kraus put JFK through his exercises. Between October 1961 and his assassination in 1963, Dr. Kraus personally attended JFK at least once or twice a week in 1961 and 1962. He attended less often in 1963 when JFK improved. He had JFK do exercises as well as swim almost daily. Dr. Kraus initially prescribed and oversaw muscle strengthening. Within six weeks the White House doctors saw an improvement and were pleasantly surprised and thankful. Their President could carry on!

Apparently, Dr. Kraus tipped off the press about JFK's early success. On December 14, 1961, the New York Times reported, "President's Back Reported Better. Back apparently is tremendously better. About six weeks ago, New York expert Dr. Hans Kraus, began coming to the White House to supervise a series of muscle strengthening exercises. Dr. Kraus still makes the visit once or twice a week. Presidential aides said he has done wonders for the President."

Dr. Kraus' treatment contained some interesting and apparently beneficial components. He removed the padding from JFK's rocking chair because he believed a hard surface would help his buttock muscles. Dr. Kraus didn't use procaine but lidocaine and occasionally gave JFK what is called a trigger point injection. A trigger point is a spot, that on feel, is taught and painful. Dr. Kraus would inject a syringe filled with lidocaine. When the needle hit the painful spot, he would twist the needle to break up scars and adhesions. This procedure is in use today and is called "dry needling." Just how many or how often he injected trigger points is unknown.

He taught JFK to do what he called K-W (Kraus-Weber) exercises. The exercises were to strengthen postural muscles that hold a person upright. Put another way, are you strong enough to effectively support your own body weight? In Susan E. B. Schwartz' enjoyable biography of Dr. Kraus, the K-W exercises that he taught JFK are shown. They are reprinted here, word-for-word, as they were the basis of JFK's most effective strength and muscle-building program.

As with any long-term medical treatment, JFKs was not straight uphill. Some days and weeks were better than others. Within about 90 days after starting his physical exercise program, JFK could do ten sit-ups with knees straight. He could bend over and touch his legs below his knees which he could not do at Dr. Kraus' initial physical examination. JFK continued to improve, and by late 1962, Dr. Kraus saw JFK only once a week. Dr. Kraus trained the White House physical therapist, "Chief" Hendrix in the K-W exercises. Mr. Hendrix traveled with JFK and saw to it he faithfully did his daily exercises.

By May of 1963, JFK felt he was well enough to resume playing golf for the first time in about two years. Dr. Kraus wasn't happy about it, because he didn't believe golf to be a "real" exercise, and worse, it might cause stress and strain on his back muscles. Dr. Kraus admonished JFK, "A couple of holes would be okay, but avoid driving practice."

The press learned of JFK's return to the golf course. On July 6, 1963 the New York Times wrote:

"Ever since May 1961...John F. Kennedy has stayed off the golf course. So it came as a surprise when, early this month, newsmen spotted the President swinging vigorously away on the course at Hyannisport...To help his ailing back, Kennedy has for two years been doing special calisthenics under the guidance

of Dr. Hans Kraus, a Vienna-trained New York physician who thinks that much back trouble is related to muscle weakness. On his recent trip to Europe, Kennedy noted how greatly his back had improved in the course of those two years. He endured the jostling and the strenuous pace without noticing any pain, and upon his return he exultantly told friends that his back was no longer troubling him. With Dr. Kraus's O.K., he decided to take up golf again. Last week at Hyannisport, he got out on the course again and swung away."

JFK continued to progressively improve although he developed two trigger points in the fall of 1963 which Dr. Kraus eliminated. At the time of the trigger points JFK asked Dr. Kraus if he should return to crutches. The answer was a firm "no" because Dr. Kraus felt supports of any kind would cause muscle atrophy. In fact, Dr. Kraus felt it was time for JFK to give up wearing his corset. JFK had worn a corset or brace since his college days at Harvard when he injured his back. Finally, in October of 1963, incidentally the last time Dr. Kraus saw JFK, he agreed to give up the corset in the upcoming new year (1964). Dr. Kraus also felt JFK didn't need the rigors of the K-W exercise program and that he should begin a maintenance exercise program of three times a week weightlifting, stretching, sit ups, pull ups, and jogging.

JFK wore his corset on the day of his assassination. Dr. M. T. Jenkins, one of the Parkland Memorial Hospital doctors who tended JFK after he was shot, described it as a tightly laced brace, held in place by wide ace bandages making figure eight loops around his torso and thighs. Many writers and historians feel the corset may have inadvertently caused JFK's death. Robert Dallek detailed in his exquisite 2002 biography, "Kennedy, An Unfinished Life" concluded, "were it not for a back brace, which held him erect, a third fatal shot to the back of the head would not have found its mark."

An irony of JFK's medical saga is that his overall health in 1963, at the time of his assassination, was probably the best in his adult life. For some time, he had been under medical and hormonal care provided by Drs. Travell and Cohen. Even Dr. Jacobson's cocktail which contained growth hormones, particularly HCG, appeared to contribute to his improved health. Admiral (Dr.) Burkley saw to it that JFK's disparate group of doctors did their job. Dr. Kraus put the "icing on the cake" with his demanding and effective physical therapy. On the last day of his life, JFK declared to one of his aides, Kenneth O'Donnell, "I feel great. My back feels better than it's felt in years." Evelyn Lincoln, JFK's secretary wrote to Dr. Kraus about twenty years after the assassination. In her letter she stated, "I have often stated that in the past six months of President Kennedy's life he was in the best health he had ever been."

To this day, few persons are aware that Dr. Kraus pulled JFK out of a disabling health hole that would have prevented him from carrying out his Presidential duties. JFK's other doctors simply had no solution to his disabling back pain. The procaine injections that initially relieved his pain and previously kept him functioning not only didn't work anymore but were probably causing his back to deteriorate into a state of weakness and immobility. Some of Dr. Kraus' regular patients described him as a "miracle worker" which is a label that could easily be applied to his treatment of JFK.

THE K-W TESTS AND EXERCISES DEVELOPED AND PRESCRIBED TO JFK BY DR. HANS KRAUS

1. Hip flexor K-W Strength Test

Lie flat on your back on the floor, hand clasped behind your neck, legs straight and touching. Keeping your knees straight, lift your feet so that your heels are ten inches above the floor. **You pass if you: Hold position for ten seconds.**

2. Hip Flexor and Stomach Muscles K-W Strength Test

Lie flat on the floor, hands clasped behind your neck. Have someone hold down your legs by grasping your ankles; or if you are by yourself, you can hook your ankles under a heavy chair that won't topple. **You pass if you: Do one sit-up.**

3. **Stomach Muscle K-W Strength Test**

Lie flat on the floor, hands behind your neck, knees flexed, heels close to your buttocks. Make sure your ankles are held down, as in exercise #2. **You pass if you: Roll up into sitting position once.**

4. **Back Muscles K-W Strength Test**

Lie on your stomach, pillow under your abdomen, clasp your hands behind your neck, lying flat on the floor. Have someone hold lower half of your body steady by placing one hand on the small of your back, the other on your ankles). Lift your trunk. **You pass if you: Hold steady for ten seconds.**

5. **Low-Back Muscles K-W Strength Test**

On your stomach, fold your arms under your head; make sure there is a pillow under your abdomen. Have someone hold your back steady with both hands. Lift your legs up, keeping your knees straight. **You pass if you: Hold position ten seconds.**

6. **Back Muscles and Ham-Strings K-W Flexibility Test**

Stand up straight, feet together. Relax, lean over, and try to touch the floor with your fingertips without bending your knees. **You pass is you: Touch the floor. NOTE*** If you fail:** It is because these muscles are shortened and tense. It is not because your arms are too short or your legs too long!

The above Table is found in "Into the Unknown: The Remarkable Life of Hans Kraus" by Susan E. B. Schwwartz, pages 265-266.

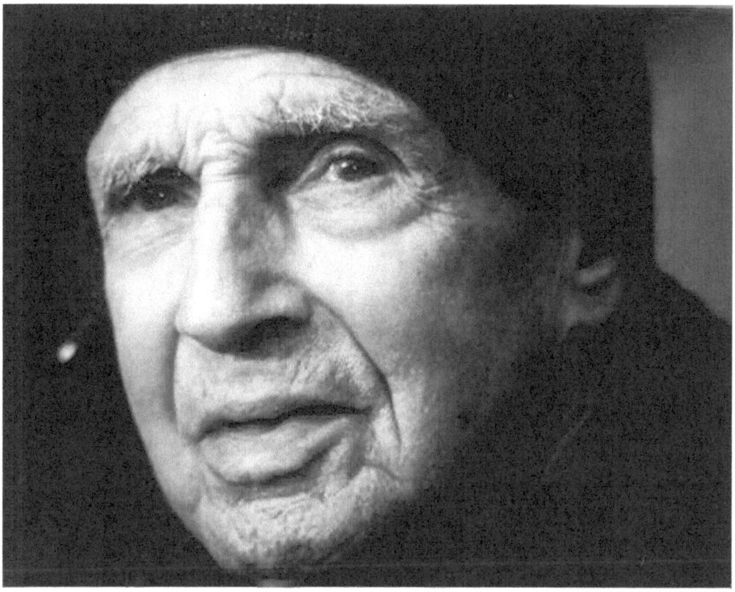

Dr. Hans Kraus expertly rehabilitated JFK's back when his longstanding prior treatments failed to bring adequate pain relief. He was an accomplished rock climber.

15. Underlying Diseases

Rare Causes of Misery

The strange medical saga of JFK began the day he was born. As stated in earlier chapters he had only one obvious physical defect at birth, which was a shortened leg. During childhood his physicians diagnosed an "unstable back." His underlying genetic disease wasn't physically visible but was far more disastrous. He had a very rare genetic disease called "autoimmune polyglandular syndrome," hereafter called APS. In simple terms, it means that an autoimmune process inside the body will "rust" and demolish glands such as the pancreas, thyroid and adrenals. The autoimmune process may also attack and rust away other tissues such as gastrointestinal tract, spine, and prostate all of which occurred in JFK.[2,7,8,11,17,18,26,27,37,38]

Adrenal hormones of which the best known is cortisone are necessary to control infections. Within a few months after birth, he started a string of infections that were essentially continuous in his childhood and early teenage years. Besides the usual childhood infections, he had a near death case of scarlet fever before age three. During his Presidency and before his assassination he had a chronic urinary – prostate infection that required almost constant antibiotics. Although his multiple medical disorders including Addison's disease, back pain, colitis, and thyroid deficiency may seem disparate and unconnected, they were all elements of his APS. Unfortunately, this disease was neither recognized nor understood for over three decades after JFK's death.

Beginning in 2002 the John F. Kennedy Presidential Library and Museum allowed researchers and historians to review what medical records of JFK they had collected after his death. Other medical records of JFK were either kept private by the many medical practitioners seen by him over the years or they were lost for review.

On three occasions in 2008, Dr. Lee R. Mandel, a US Naval endocrinologist, was permitted to review JFK's medical records three times at the Presidential Museum. After his review, he astutely and expertly determined that JFK was genetically born with the rare disease known as, "Autoimmune Polyendocrine Syndrome Type II (APS)."[19] Dr. Mandel clearly "hit the nail on the head" in analyzing the underlying cause of JFK's medical saga. He published his findings in the prestigious medical journal, "Annals of Internal Medicine" in 2009. The William's Textbook of Endocrinology, 14th edition (2020) is considered in medical circles the "bible" of endocrinology. It defines APS as "the occurrence in the same patient of two or more of the following: primary adrenal insufficiency (Addison's disease), Grave's disease, autoimmune thyroiditis, diabetes, primary hypogonadism, myasthenia gravis, and celiac disease. Vitiligo, alopecia, serositis, and pernicious anemia also occur with increased frequency in patients with this syndrome and in their family members." There are two types of APS, the difference between APS Type I and II is that Type I does not have celiac disease. As described in previous chapters JFK began crippling abdominal symptoms starting at about age ten. Symptoms included intermittent nausea, vomiting, bloating, pain, and alternating diarrhea and constipation.[2] Today's term for this medical entity, celiac disease, didn't come into play until after the death of JFK. For example, the 1962 Dorland's Medical Dictionary doesn't list the term celiac disease.[9] JFK was, therefore, given various terms for his intestinal disease which included "duodenitis" and "colitis."

APS was first described in 1926 by a German pathologist, Dr. M. B. Schmidt.[29] Physicians, sometimes call the combination of adrenal and thyroid insufficiency, "Schmidt's Syndrome."[8] JFK well fits the definition of APS Type II. His endocrine disease attacked three glands: the adrenals, testicles, and thyroid. He eventually needed cortisone, thyroid, and testosterone replacement. Dr. Travell diagnosed pernicious anemia which is vitamin B_{12} deficiency when she took on JFK as a patient in 1955. He was 38 years old. Anemia and adrenal gland insufficiency go "hand in hand" with APS.[2,8,11,30]

Unfortunately, autoimmunity and immune deficiencies were just starting to be recognized, understood, and therapeutically treated about the time of JFK's assassination. For example, the 1962 edition of Dorland's Medical Dictionary does not even list autoimmune disease.[9] The 1965 edition of Current Therapy only refers to "autoimmune reactions."[15] Beginning in the1960's the medical profession began to accept the fact that the body may actually turn on itself. Simply, autoimmunity is defined as a biologic reaction in which the body attacks and destroys some of its own tissues. In contrast to the 1962 edition, Dorland's Medical Dictionary in 1981 defined autoimmunity as "a condition characterized by a specific humoral or cell-mediated immune response against the constituents of the body's own tissues."[10]

In a normal immune system, antibodies circulate throughout the body and immediately attack and neutralize any infectious agent, poison, or toxic substance that may enter the body. An autoimmune disease is one in which an "autoantibody" rather than "antibody" may emerge in the bloodstream and literally attack tissue in one's own body, initiate oxygenation ("rusting"), inflammation, pain, and tissue destruction.[7,11,17] JFK began incessant infections within weeks following his birth indicating that immune deficiencies had a genetic basis.

Today, many people are under the impression that JFK's PT109 incident is what led to his back and medical issues. This is only partially correct. He already had some genetic autoimmune disease deterioration in his spine prior to his Naval service. The PT109 incident clearly exacerbated his condition because he didn't have an adequate immune system to fight and control the stress of his ordeal. His back pain worsened after the PT109 incident and this led to his first back surgery in 1944 as well as his discharge from the Navy within a year.

Besides APS, there was a second rare disease that, in retrospect, appeared to cause much, if not most, of his unbearable back pain.

Dr. Charles Burton who, in a forty-year career, served as a professor at Johns Hopkins and Temple University. In his later life, he founded the Department of Neuroaugmentive Surgery at the Sister Kenny Institute in Minneapolis, Minnesota. In his work as a neurosurgeon, he became aware of the rare disease called "adhesive arachnoiditis" (AA). In September 2019, he published a medical report entitled, "Adhesive Arachnoiditis: The Day They Poisoned JFK."[6] Dr. Burton and Dr. Antonio Aldrete, an anesthesiologist, discovered that the dye used in spinal myelograms in the 1940's can cause AA. The agent was called Pantopaque® in the USA and Myodil® in Europe. These dyes were sometimes toxic and irritating to the cauda equina nerve roots that are suspended in the lower (lumbar-sacral) portion of the spinal canal. The toxic and irritating property of the dye, which is insoluble in spinal fluid, could sometimes cause inflammation in the cauda equina nerve roots. Once inflamed they formed adhesions that resulted in an entrapped mass of nerve roots inside the spinal canal. The inflamed mass glued the nerve roots to the inside lining of the spinal canal covering which is called the arachnoid membrane. Hence the name "adhesive arachnoiditis (AA)." This disorder was first identified and defined in 1873 as "inflammation of the arachnoid membrane." During the 1800's it was sometimes called the "devil's disease." It may cause the worst of all pain and lead to immense disability and suffering. JFK could be the "poster child" for AA as his symptoms and wish to die rather than endure the pain is typical of the disease. Although the incidence and prevalence of AA after a Pantopaque® myelogram is unknown, Dr. Aldrete felt it occurred often enough that in 2003 he labeled the Pantopaque® issue "The Silent Epidemic."

Dr. Burton made the determination that JFK had AA after he saw an x-ray taken by the British physician, Sir Daniel Davis, who diagnosed JFK's Addison's disease is 1947. This x-ray was taken by Harley Laboratories in London on October 7, 1947, and later released to Julian's Auction. It was revealed on an internet site called "X-rays of Famous People" which was initially accessed on May 22, 2015. The x-ray is shown here. It clearly shows that Pantopaque® dye is still in the spinal canal. The dye was obviously injected into JFK's spinal fluid by another party prior to 1947 or it may have been done by Dr. Davis to better determine what pathologic conditions may exist in JFK's spinal canal. Regardless, Dr. Burton believed that entrapment of the toxic dye had to cause AA. Pantopaque®, not only contributed to or caused most of JFK's pain, it also provides a reason why JFK didn't benefit from two major back surgeries. For example, Dr. James Poppen, the neurosurgeon at the Lahey Clinic who performed JFK's first major back surgery on June 23, 1944, didn't have an explanation for the surgery's failure. His apologetic statement regarding the surgery is found in Chapter Ten.

It is noted in Dr. Poppen's note that JFK's L5-S1 disc was abnormally soft and that the posterior ligament was firmly adhered to the nerve root. The soft disc material suggests on-going autoimmune deterioration and the ligament-nerve root adherence had to be by adhesions. This descriptive note suggests that autoimmunity and AA were already in place and possibly responsible for the surgical failure. The second major back surgery, in 1954, may also have failed because his pain and need for crutches was due to AA and not an anatomic defect that could be helped by surgery.

In Dr. Burton's report, he claims Pantopaque® was never officially approved for use in myelograms and that perhaps hundreds of military personnel were injected with Pantopaque® dye without their knowledge beginning in 1942. The report also claims that another neurosurgeon, Dr. William Van Wagenen, recognized in 1943 that Pantopaque® caused inflammation and a "chemical meningitis". Apparently, this finding wasn't definitive enough to discontinue Pantopaque® use. Its use in the 1940's and 50's led to AA and infrequently led to early death. The complications of Pantopaque® eventually forced its discontinuation as a myelographic dye. It was, consequently, replaced by safer dyes. Magnetic resonance imaging was invented in about 1987 which obviated the use of Pantopaque®.

AA causes dysfunction in the nerve connection between the spinal cord and the bladder, intestine, and legs. Chronic urinary infections and symptoms of colitis are common with AA. Severe back pain and the need for back braces and crutches is routinely required with AA. Suicide is common. It is possible that JFK's chronic urinary tract infection and colitis symptoms were initially caused by APS and then aggravated by AA.

In summary, JFK was born with a rare genetic, autoimmune disease called "Autoimmune Polyglandular Syndrome". It was complicated by the development of another rare disease called "adhesive arachnoiditis" which was caused by myelogram dye called Pantopaque® injected into his spinal canal during the early 1940's. All of his myriad medical conditions can be explained by these two conditions. Unfortunately, JFK's physicians could only treat the symptoms of the two underlying causes of his maladies because medical science had neither identified nor understood these two rare diseases during the lifetime of JFK.

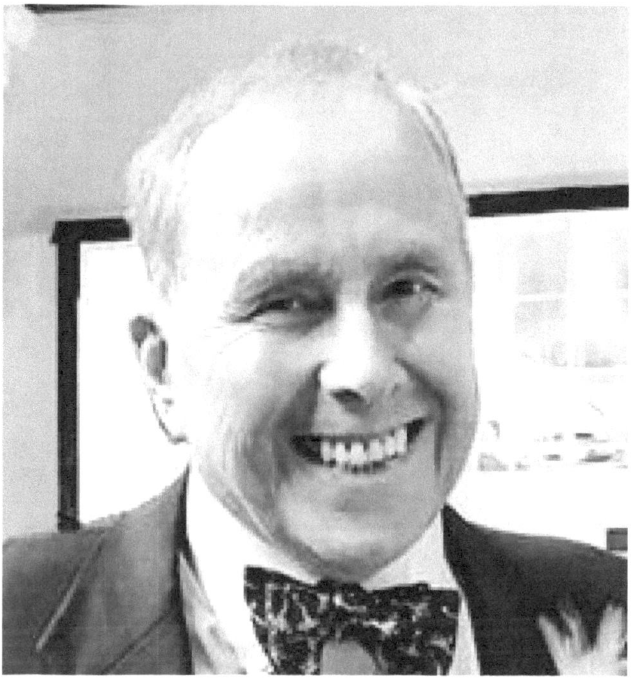

Dr. Charles V. (Chuck) Burton was a renowned neurosurgeon who determined that JFK developed adhesive arachnoiditis that contributed to his intractable back pain.

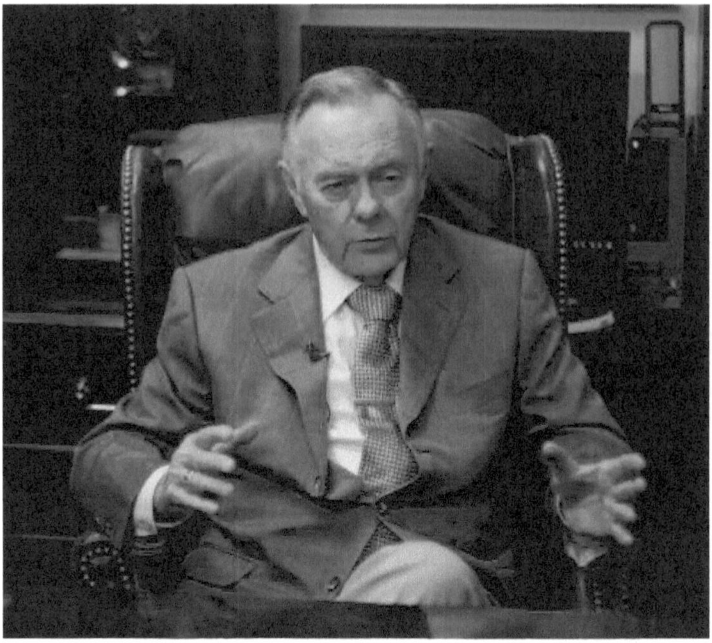

Dr. Lee Mandell was a US Naval endocrinologist who determined that JFK had a rare genetic autoimmune endocrine disease which was the basic cause of his lifetime health problems.

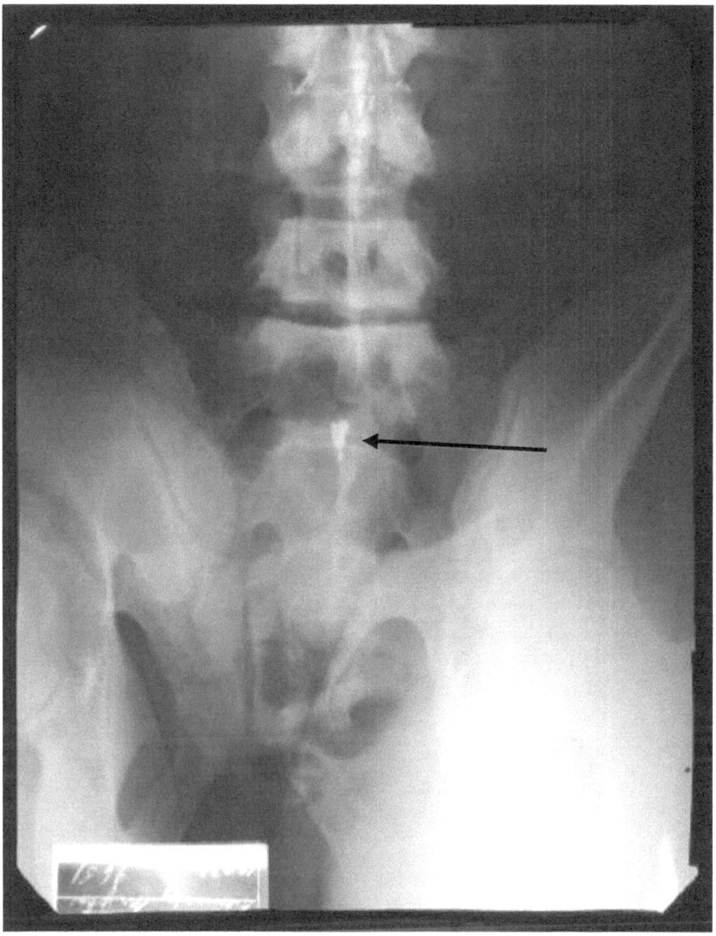

X-ray of JFK shows that myelogram dye (Pantopaque®) is in the spinal canal long after it was injected.

16. Assassination and Autopsy: November 1963 (Age 46)

Addison's Disease Confirmed

JFK was assassinated on November 22, 1963, at the age of 46. After his assassination, and until this day, there is argument and controversy over the number of bullets that killed JFK as well as the direction from which the bullets were fired. This translates to whether the bullets entered his head and body from the front or back. A Federal Commission called the Warren Commission investigated the assassination and reviewed JFK's autopsy that was done at the Bethesda Naval Hospital. The Warren Commission Report concluded that a lone assassin named Lee Harvey Oswald fired two shots that entered JFK from the rear, causing death. Since 1963, however, some parties have not accepted this conclusion.

In an attempt to clarify the issue, the physicians in the emergency department at Dallas Parkland Hospital, where JFK was taken in a futile effort to save him, have spoken out. Four doctors were the principals who treated JFK at Parkland. Dr. Malcolm Perry, who did the tracheotomy; Dr. Jim Carrico, a surgical resident, the first to treat JFK and who observed that an exit wound was on the front of his neck before the tracheotomy; Dr. MT "Pepper" Jenkins, chief of Anesthesiology, who attempted to ventilate JFK, and Dr. Charles Baxter, a surgeon who assisted in the resuscitation attempt. All four of these physicians have emphasized that two bullets entered JFK from the rear and caused his death.

Despite the claims of the Parkland Hospital physicians and the Warren Commission, there were strenuous rejections of the "two bullets from the rear" conclusion in many circles for some time after his death. In 1992, 29 years after JFK's death, Dr. George Lundberg, a former military pathologist and editor of the Journal of the American Medical Association, attempted to bring resolution and finalization to the argument. He enlisted the most renowned medical journalist of the time, Dennis L. Breo, to assist him. Dr. Lundberg and Mr. Breo contended that only two physicians could tell the public precisely the facts. These were the US Naval pathologists who did JFK's autopsy. Dr. Lundberg and Mr. Breo arranged to extensively interview these two pathologists in April 1992. Prior to this time the two pathologists had made scant remarks about the autopsy.

JFK was pronounced dead at 1:00 PM on November 22, 1963, at Dallas' Parkland Hospital. He, along with Jackie Kennedy and Admiral George Burkley, the White House Physician, boarded Air Force One for a flight back to Washington. Admiral, Dr. Burkley called the Armed Forces Institute of Pathology (AFIP). It was considered the pinnacle of military pathology and perhaps world pathology. It was generally assumed that JFK's autopsy would be done at AFIP, but during the flight, Jackie Kennedy requested that an autopsy be done, and that it be done at the Bethesda National Naval Medical Center. Dr. Humes, who headed the autopsy team, later stated that Mrs. Kennedy selected the Naval Hospital since her husband had been a Navy man.

On the day the President was shot at 12:30 PM, while riding in an open motorcade through the sunny streets of Dallas, Texas, it was cold and gray in the Washington, DC area. US Naval Commander James Joseph Humes, MC then 39, was the director of labs of the Naval Medical School in Bethesda, MD. US Naval Commander J. Thornton Boswell, MC, then 41, was Chief of Pathology at the Naval Hospital. Dr. Humes was Dr. Boswell's boss.

At about 5:15 PM on November 22, 1963, Dr. Humes was home helping his wife prepare for a dinner party. He received an emergency call from the Surgeon General of the Navy, Admiral Edward Denney. He succinctly said, "Jim, you better hurry over to the hospital." By the time he reached the hospital within the hour, he entered and Admiral Kenney, the ranking military officer said, "to be prepared to do an autopsy on the late President." Dr. Humes stated that his orders were to find the cause of death and, "I was told to get anyone I thought necessary to help do the autopsy, but to limit it to only the help I needed. Hell, I could have called in people from Paris and Rome if I thought it necessary."

By 7:30 PM Dr. Humes was in his scrubs. He selected Dr. Boswell as his assistant as he knew he had top talent at his fingertips.

When Drs. Humes and Boswell opened JFK's casket to begin a four-hour autopsy, they saw the devastating nature of his head wound. Dr. Humes then communicated with Dr. Bruce Smith, the deputy director of the Armed Forces Institute of Pathology. Initially Dr. Humes thought he might need the assistance of an expert neuropathologist, but the head wound was so large and such an obvious cause of death that Dr. Smith sent an expert in ballistics named Dr. Pierre A. Finck. He was a shy retiring man who was an army colonel. He arrived about 9:15 PM to complete the team of three who are credited for doing JFK's autopsy.

The complete autopsy took around four hours, until about midnight. Drs. Humes and Boswell remained in the morgue until 5:00 AM the next morning helping to embalm the President's body. Dr. Humes reported that, "we were able to almost perfectly restore the President's appearance and a local funeral home brought out a beautiful mahogany casket to replace the bronze one from Dallas."

Dr. Burkley and Robert and Jackie Kennedy took JFK in the new casket to the White House. The next task was to prepare an autopsy report which Dr. Burkley wanted within forty-eight hours. Being an Admiral and a doctor, he had the authority to demand this action which was carried out.

The main component of Drs. Humes and Boswell's report is stated below. Dr. Lundberg and Mr. Breo's interview with the two doctors was summarized in the May 27, 1992, issue of the Journal of American Medical Association. They were adamant in their conclusion:

"The evidence produced in the four-hour autopsy at Bethesda Naval Hospital provides irrefutable proof that the President was struck by only two bullets that came from above and behind from a high velocity weapon which caused the fatal wound."

Although the Lundberg-Breo report was intended primarily to resolve controversy surrounding the assassination, they also revealed that JFK's autopsy showed almost zero adrenal tissue. This settled the longstanding dispute as to whether he did or did not have Addison's disease. The adrenal glands did not show any cancerous or infectious infiltration such as tuberculosis or syphilis. This finding supported autoimmunity as the cause of his Addison's Disease. In 1992 a book entitled, "High Treason II." claimed that the pathologists who did the autopsy could not find the adrenals, despite careful serial sections of the perirenal fat. No mention of the adrenals was given to the Warren Commission likely because it was only interested in his cause of death and not his medical issues. The first public statement about the lack of adrenal glands at autopsy was provided to "High Treason" by Robert F. Carnei, MD, who was a pathology resident at the Bethesda Naval Hospital at the time of JFK's death. He had observed firsthand that no adrenal tissue could be grossly found on routine dissection.

Dr. Lundberg was, in contrast to the Warren Commission, extremely interested in whether JFK had Addison's disease. After all, in 1992 there had been about a 30-year public debate over whether he did or did not have Addison's. Here is Dr. Lundberg and Mr. Breo's conclusion:[4,16]

"On August 31, 1992, Dr. Boswell confirmed, on the record, that serial sections of the perirenal fat pads demonstrated no gross evidence of adrenal cortex or medulla. Microscopically, Dr. Boswell found a few individual adrenal cortical cells immersed in a sea of fat. There was no scarring, inflammation, or granuloma formation. This observation, along with the clinical evidence is diagnostic of severe Addison's disease, which is not of tuberculous origin."

In summary, although there may today still be some disagreement over the number of bullets and direction from which they were fired, the physicians who tried to save him at Dallas Parkland Hospital and who did his autopsy at the Bethesda Naval Hospital are in agreement. He was killed by two bullets shot from the rear. Dr. George Lundberg and Mr. Dennis Breo, both known personally to this author as honest, credible professionals, interviewed and published the experiences and autopsy findings of pathologists Drs. James Humes and J. T. Boswell. They both forcefully opine that JFK was killed by two bullets from the rear. Besides an attempt to close arguments as to the case of JFK's cause of death, Dr. Lundberg and Mr. Breo were able to confirm that JFK's adrenal glands were essentially nonexistent at autopsy. This finding fully supports the notion that JFK had Addison's disease caused by autoimmunity and not tuberculosis.

<u>Original November 24, 1963, Autopsy Report</u>

"The fatal missile entered the skull above and to the right of the external occipital protuberance. A portion of the projectile traversed the cranial cavity in a posterior-anterior direction (see lateral skull roentgenograms), depositing minute particles along its path. A portion of the projectile made its exit through the parietal bone on the right, carrying with it portions of cerebrum, skull, and scalp. The two wounds of the skull combined with the force of the missile produced extensive fragmentation of the skull, laceration of the superior sagittal alnus, and the right cerebral hemisphere.

The other missile entered the right superior posterior thorax above the scapula and traversed the soft tissue of the supra-scapular and supra-clavicular portions of the base of the right side of the neck. This missile produced contusions of the right apical parietal pleura and of the apical portion of the right upper lobe of the lung. The missile contused the strap muscles of the right side of the neck, damaged the trachea, and made its exit through the anterior surface of the neck. As far as can be ascertained, this missile struck no bony structures in its path through the body.

In addition, it is our opinion that the wound of the skull produces such extensive damage to the brain as to preclude the possibility of the deceased surviving this injury.

It is our opinion that the deceased died as a result of two perforating gunshot wounds inflicted by high-velocity projectiles fired by a person or persons unknown. The projectiles were fired from a point behind and somewhat above the level of the deceased. The observation and available information do not permit a satisfactory estimate as to the sequence of the two wounds.

A supplementary report will be submitted following more detailed examinations of the brain and of microscopic sections. However, it is not anticipated that these examinations will materially alter the findings."

Supplementary report submitted on December 6, 1963.

"This supplementary report covers in more detail the extensive degree of cerebral trauma in this case. However, neither this portion of the examination nor the microscopic examination alter the previously submitted report or add significant details to the cause of death."

This report was signed by Drs. Humes, Boswell, and Finck and submitted to Dr. Admiral George Burkley, the White House Chief Physician.

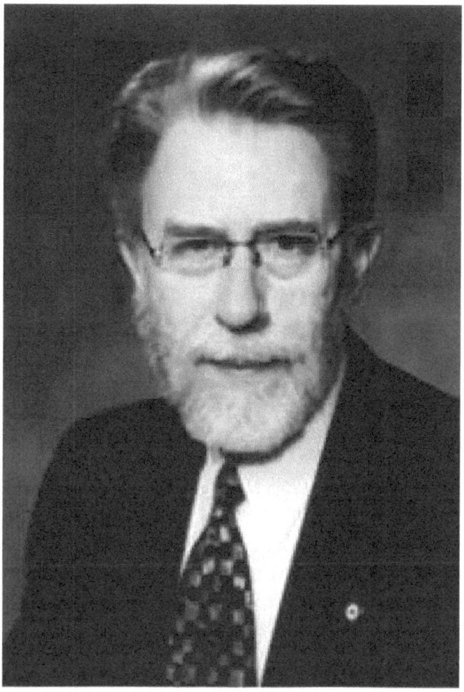

Dr. George Lundberg was a former military pathologist and editor of the Journal of American Medical Association. He brought together the pathologists who did JFK's autopsy to clarify that two bullets fired from the rear killed JFK and that he definitely had Addison's disease.

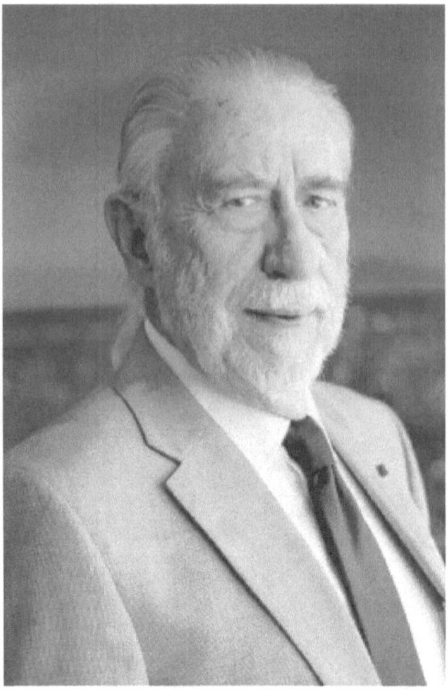

Dennis Breo, noted medical journalist, who worked with Dr. George Lundberg to document the cause of JFK's death and determined whether he truly had Addison's disease.

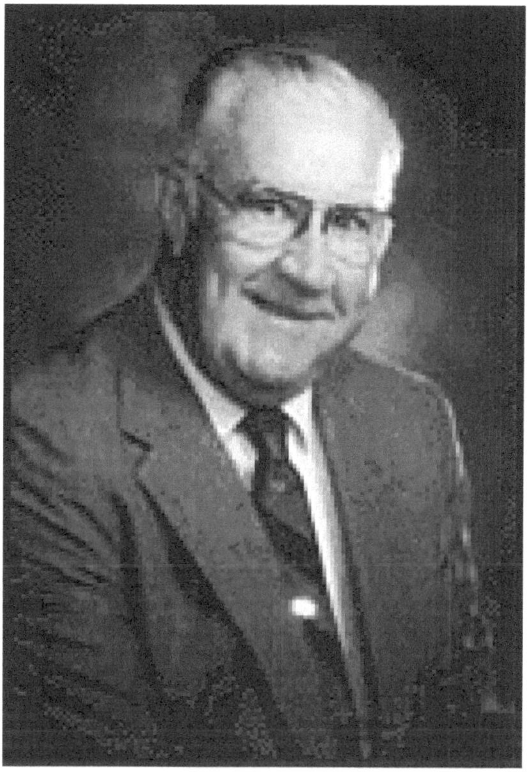

Dr. James Humes was the US Naval Commander and pathologist who led the team that did JFK's autopsy at the US Naval Bethesda Hospital.

17. The Medical Cover Up

A Public Necessity

On July 5, 1960, just about four months before JFK's Presidential election, his two main physicians, Dr. Janet Travell and Eugene J. Cohen, sent a signed letter to JFK for public dissemination. The letter was specifically designed to let the public know that Senator Kennedy was fit enough for the Presidency. The letter stated, *"As your physicians for over five years and with knowledge of your medical records for over 15 years, we wish to provide you with a straightforward, brief medical statement concerning your health. As stated to you in our recent letter of 6/11/60 we reiterate that you are in superb physical condition – you should see your doctors once or twice a year for a routine check-up – no limitations are placed on your arduous activities."*

This letter was distributed to the press. It appeared to be well accepted at the time. JFK was tall, trim, and affable. This author, as a junior college student, actually met JFK during his primary campaign in 1960 when he and Hubert Humphrey, two of the Presidential Democrat contenders, came to Hutchinson, Kansas Community college to debate. JFK did not appear to be ill. He was vivacious, energetic, and did not appear to be ill. We loved him! The letter above, however, later became generally known as a blatant cover up for his ill health. There is little question that a part of JFK's strange medical saga is that his family and political handlers went to great length to keep the public from knowing his true medical history. They obviously believed that the election could be lost if the public became aware of his true health issues. He had been given last rites on two occasions, had two failed major back surgeries, and required a complex medical program including methadone and other opioids to carry out normal activities of daily living. What his doctors did not know was that autoimmunity was the cause of his Addison's Disease rather than tuberculosis.

The letter written by Drs. Travell and Cohen had its aegis by claims from JFK's political opponents in early 1960, who believed he had Addison's disease. At that point in history, Addison's disease was still perceived as being caused by tuberculosis. While about 90% of cases in the 1800's may have been caused by tuberculosis, by the middle of the 1900's, anti-tuberculosis drugs had been developed and had eliminated this infection as a major cause of Addison's. The medical profession wasn't yet aware of this as autoimmunity wasn't even medically recognized as an initiator of any disease. In addition to Drs. Travell and Cohen's letter, Robert Kennedy, and a family representative, provided this statement to the press and public just before the November 1960 election.

"John F. Kennedy has not, nor has he ever, had an ailment described classically as Addison's disease, which is a tuberculous destruction of the adrenal gland. Any statement to the contrary is malicious and false...In the post-war period he had some mild adrenal insufficiency, and this is not in any way a dangerous condition. And it is possible that even this might be corrected over the years since ACTH stimulation tests for adrenal function were considered normal in 1958. Doctors

have stated that this condition might have arisen out of his wartime experiences of shock and malaria."

The above statement has been criticized. For example, Dr. John R. Bumgardner, in his 2004 book entitled "The Health of Presidents" stated, *"This was undoubtedly one of the most cleverly laid smokescreens ever put down around a politician."*

Dr. Bumgardner's book was on the health status of 48 Presidents, beginning with George Washington and chronologically ending with William Jefferson Clinton. JFK was included. Dr. Bumgardner makes the distinct point that a concerted effort has surrounded almost all the Presidents in US history to keep their health status a secret from the general public. JFK was no exception.

Interestingly, on July 28, 1955, the Archives of Surgery published an article by James A. Nichols and co-authors. Although JFK's name was not used in the article, an astute investigator could have easily determined who the article was about and documented that JFK had Addison's disease. The time of admission coincided with that of JFK. The description in the journal was of a 37-year-old male who had Addison's Disease for seven years, had been in treatment with DOCA implants, 150 mg for three months, and cortisone 25 mg by mouth daily. Orthopedic consultation suggested that he might be helped by lumbosacral and sacroiliac fusion. Dr. Ephraim Shorr, an endocrinologist at New York Hospital, provided advice in the management of the case. The operation was done on October 21, 1954, the same day as JFK's surgery.

JFK's family and political handlers weren't apparently eager to reveal anything that might be perceived as negative about his health. The denial of Addison's disease or other health issues didn't prevent JFK from being elected President in November 1960. During the campaign JFK was portrayed as someone who was young, healthy, and had vigor (JFK pronounced this last term "vigah"). On his inauguration day, January 20, 1961, it was freezing cold. While everyone in the crowd was bundled with coats, hats, scarves, and gloves, to "prove his good health" JFK gave his acceptance speech in just his suit without hat, coat, scarf, or gloves.

After JFK was elected, secrecy about his health issues continued. Dr. Edward MacMahon and Leonard Curry authored a book in 1987 entitled, "Medical Cover-Ups in the White House." They described the secrecy that surrounded his use of multiple medications including opioids and cortisone as well as the conflicts between his physicians. They emphasized that treatment by Dr. Max Jacobson was kept as secret as possible. Attached is an Enquirer Magazine ad of the type commonly portrayed to denigrate JFK after he died.

Maintaining secrecy about medical issues involving a sitting President who must deal with threats of war and nuclear attack is a judgement call. The Kennedy family hardly revealed any health information about JFK during his presidency and did not allow journalists or physician researchers to review his medical records until 2002. Although health secrecy for Presidents is understandable, the Kennedy family, his doctors, and his political handlers had another problem. How could they explain the myriad of health problems such as the two "last rites" episodes that befell him? They had no idea about his causative diseases of autoimmunity and arachnoiditis.

Despite secrecy or cover-ups, JFK's overall health improved after Dr. Travell took over his care in 1955 and during his 1000 days in the White House. His four main doctors, Travell, Jacobson, Kraus and Cohen independently administered separate therapeutic programs that had a combined positive effect. Dr. Admiral Burkley kept all of JFK's innovative doctors working as a rather miraculous team to make sure that the Presidency was well executed. Given the rarity of JFK's diseases and the innovative, unusual nature of his treatments, an argument can well be made that secrecy was a good thing.

In summary, in the months just prior to his assassination JFK's pain had reduced and his strength and energy had improved. His health and treatments were kept secret, but JFK progressively improved his health after he entered the White House. His overall health in the year he died was the best in his life. In addition, his health may have continued to improve if he had not met an untimely death. Although the secrecy surrounding his health has been highly condemned, JFK functioned well, thanks to his excellent medical care.

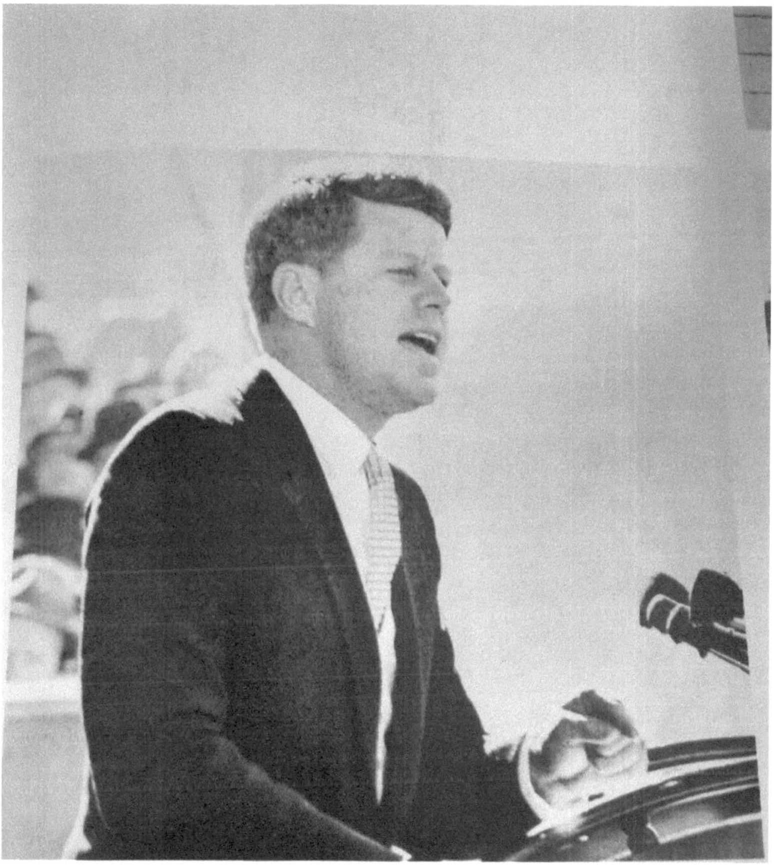

In freezing weather on inauguration day, January 20, 1960, JFK spoke without a coat or hat to give an image of good health.

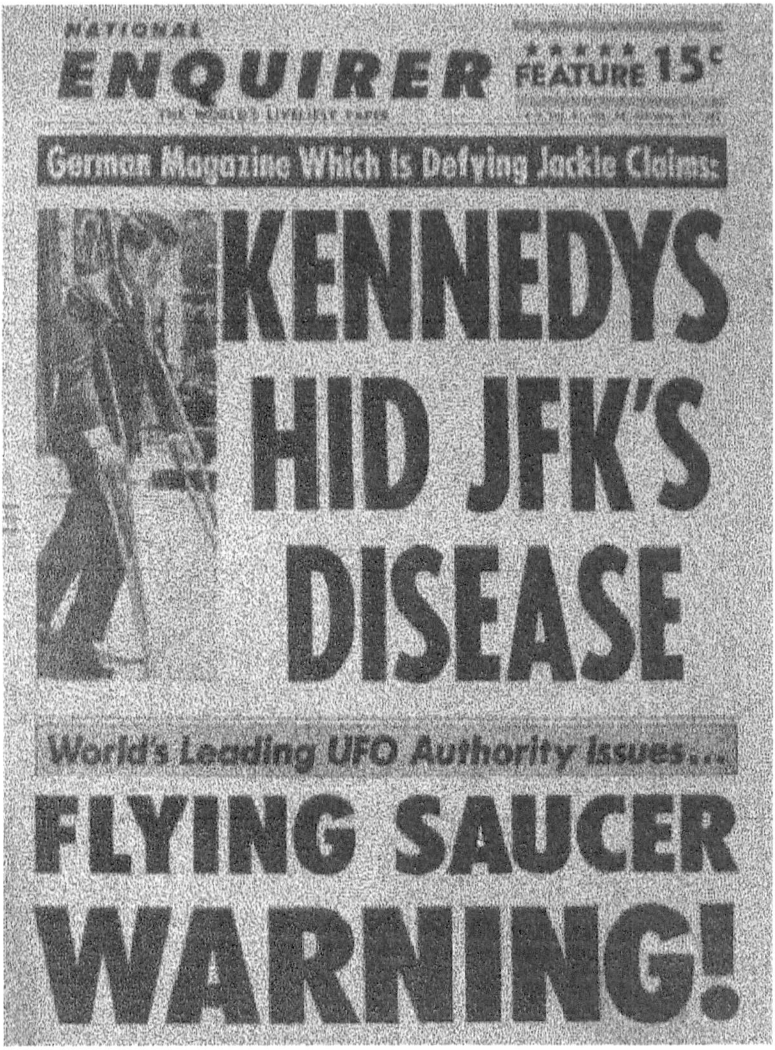
NATIONAL ENQUIRER

FEATURE 15¢

German Magazine Which Is Defying Jackie Claims:

KENNEDYS HID JFK'S DISEASE

World's Leading UFO Authority Issues...

FLYING SAUCER WARNING!

Typical claim about JFK's health issues after he died.

18. The Amazing Attitude of JFK

A Drive to Live

An amazing aspect of JFK's medical saga was his attitude about his infirmities and disease. Most people with his diseases would be bitter and hostile. Not JFK. Throughout his many ordeals, there was never any public acknowledgement of his ailments and never was there an indication of outward self-pity. He used a biting sense of humor to carry him through. He refused to let his health issues stop him from pursuing his political career.

Both JFK's brother, Robert, and longtime political advisor, Theodore Sorenson, gave statements that clearly describe his attitudes and beliefs about his health. In Robert Kennedy's book, "As We Remember Him." he wrote:

"At least one half of the days that he spent on this earth were days of intense physical pain. He had scarlet fever when he was very young and serious back trouble when he was older. In between he had almost every other conceivable ailment. When

we were growing up together, we used to laugh about the great risk a mosquito took in biting Jack Kennedy – with some of his blood the mosquito was almost sure to die.

I never heard him complain. I never heard him say anything that would indicate that he felt God had dealt with him unjustly. Those who know him well would know he was suffering only because his face was a little whiter, the lines around his eyes were a little deeper, his words a little sharper. Those who did not know him well detected nothing".

Ted Sorenson, his close adviser since 1953, struck a similar theme in describing JFK's health problems during his later life. "Never complaining about his pains or imagining new ones," Mr. Sorensen wrote in his book, Kennedy: The Classic Biography, "he used (and carried with him about the country) more pills, potions, poultices and other paraphernalia than would be found in a small dispensary." The point Mr. Sorensen sought to stress was that JFK never permitted medical difficulties to stop him from energetically and effectively performing his Presidential and political tasks. The physical ailments listed by Mr. Sorensen were formidable: allergies, poor hearing, a sensitive stomach, an old knee injury that occasionally acted up and caused him to limp as well as his major health problems which were severe pain and Addison's disease.

As a child, John Kennedy showed the effects of such illnesses as scarlet fever, diphtheria, and whooping cough. When he was fourteen, he weighed only 95 pounds and, in that year, he had to halt his studies. But unlike most children beset by chronic physical ailments, Jack did not willingly sit on the sidelines and let others compete. Even if his family had allowed him to give in to his condition, to do so was not in his nature. Despite the painful consequences, whenever he could at all physically manage it, he played football, tennis, and was an excellent sailor and swimmer.

An amazing characteristic about JFK was his humor about his health conditions. Some of his comments about his health are embarrassingly funny. For example, over the Summer of 1933, after he had turned sixteen, he gained no weight. And matters got worse the following year. In the winter of 1934, he became very sick and had to be rushed by ambulance to New Haven Hospital for observation. His symptoms included weight loss and a bad case of hives. Doctors feared that he had leukemia and began regularly checking his blood counts. "*It seems that I was much sicker than I thought I was*" JFK wrote to his classmate LeMoyne Billings after he got out of the hospital, "*and am supposed to be dead, so I am developing a limp and a hollow cough.*" His rectum was "*plenty red in the hospital,*" he complained. "*Yours would be red too if you had shoved everything from rubber tubes to iron pipes up it.*"

Six days later he gave his friend, LeMoyne, another graphic description of his ordeal. *"I've got something wrong with my intestines. In other words, I shit blood."* He feared he might be dying. The doctors were still trying to determine the cause of his illness. "*Yesterday I went through the most harassing experience of my life."* JFK wrote. *"A doctor stuck an iron tube 12 inches long and 1 inch in diameter up my ass...My poor bedraggled rectum is looking at me very reproachfully these days...The reason I'm here is that they may have to cut out my stomach!!!-the latest news."*

By the end of January 1936, he spent two months at Peter Bent Brigham Hospital. He was more worried than ever about his health, though he continued to use humor to defend himself against thoughts of dying. He wrote in a letter to LeMoyne, *"Took a peak (sic) at my chart yesterday and could see that they were mentally measuring me for a coffin. Eat, drink, and make Olive (his current girlfriend), as tomorrow or next week we attend my funeral. I think the Rockefeller Institute may take my case...Flash-they are going to stick that tube up my ass again as they did at Mayo."*

JFK exhibited another characteristic of people with severe chronic illness that tend to please and encourage physicians. Many, if not most, patients who have chronic intractable and incurable conditions sort of "give-up." take medications and succumb to a bed or house bound existence. Not JFK. He never gave up looking for and trying new treatments and medical advice. After surgical failure in 1955, he was naturally despondent but apparently didn't give up hope. When one of his physicians said he knew a physician who was an expert in pain management and back rehabilitation, he jumped at a chance to see her. Low and behold he found Dr. Travell.

His Presidential campaign understandably drained and fatigued him to the point he was afraid he couldn't compete in the nation's first televised Presidential debate. One of his close friends said there was a doctor who specialized in stress management. Dr. Max Jacobson may have been controversial, but he provided what JFK needed. Despite animosity and skirmish between his White House doctors, JFK grabbed expert medical advice whenever and wherever he could. Drs. George Burkley and Eugene Cohen told JFK that they knew just the doctor who could better his back. He brought in Dr. Hans Kraus, who was a master at muscle and strength building. His back pain reduced.

You can bet on one thing. If JFK had not been assassinated in 1963 at age 46, he would have continued searching for new and better treatments. We will, of course, never know, but I bet if JFK had lived, he would eventually have become a teacher and preacher on how to thrive and survive terrible health when the odds are stacked against you! A man who has survived "last rites" on two occasions has plenty to teach.

19. Summary

Today's public only knows that JFK had Addison's or was hurt in a PT boat. His medical saga is far more complex. He was born with a rare genetic disease which is hardly known today by physicians unless they specialize in endocrinology. His disease called "Autoimmune Polyglandular Endocrinopathy" means that the body turns on itself and wipes out glands that produce hormones such as insulin, cortisone, and thyroid. This disease has some family history as exemplified by his sister who had adrenal insufficiency. Within weeks after birth JFK began incessant infections including scarlet fever from which he was fortunate to survive. At birth he had one leg shorter than the other and some of his physicians felt he had an "unstable back." During childhood he had some joint pain. The development of back and hip pain during college continued and followed him into the US Navy. His teenage years saw the onset of gastrointestinal symptoms including diarrhea, bloating, pain, and bleeding which continued into adulthood. His condition was labeled at the time as "duodenitis" or "colitis." Today, he would be labeled as having celiac disease.

While in the Navy during World War II, he commanded a patrol torpedo boat in the South Pacific known as PT109. His boat was cut in two by a Japanese destroyer. To survive, JFK had to swim some three to five miles using a lifejacket while towing an injured sailor to an island where he and his crew were rescued. This incident exacerbated his back pain which led to major spine surgery in 1944 and a Navy discharge due to physical disability. The surgery did not relieve his pain and his doctors were mystified at the poor results.

It is likely that a myelogram using a dye called Pantopaque® was done prior to 1947. The dye is visible in an x-ray taken by Sir Daniel Davis, the British physician, who diagnosed JFK with Addison's Disease in 1947. JFK was so sick and debilitated at that time that he was given "last rites" of the Catholic faith. He was started on a cortisone derivative called deoxycorticosterone or DOCA and managed to survive. His back pain progressively worsened. It is likely that Pantopaque® dye caused a rare toxic inflammation involving the lumbar spine nerve roots. This condition is called adhesive arachnoiditis. By 1954 when he was a Senator, his pain and inability to walk had progressed to the point that he required crutches and he missed many days of work. Out of desperation he agreed to a second major back surgery in 1954. At that time he said he would rather die than go on living with his pain. Unfortunately, the surgery failed, and he appeared so terminal post-operatively that he was again given "last rights." He somehow survived but was left in severe pain. His endocrinologist sent him to Dr. Janet Travell who was perhaps the world's most renowned rehabilitation and pain specialist. She immediately hospitalized JFK and began a comprehensive medical and rehabilitation program that included methadone, procaine injections, sleep medication, and a rocking chair among other drugs and therapies. Due to her comprehensive treatment, JFK recovered to the point that he was strong enough to run for President beginning in about 1957. The campaign exhausted JFK, and in July 1960, some three to four months before the Presidential election, he consulted Dr. Max Jacobson who specialized in stress and fatigue management. Dr. Jacobson provided JFK with his own formulated cocktail whose main ingredients were methamphetamine, niacin, and human chorionic gonadotropin (HCG).

JFK was quite worried that he had to face Richard Nixon in the first televised Presidential debate in US history. On the day of the debate, he was hoarse from all his speaking engagements, and he was quite exhausted. Dr. Jacobson injected JFK's throat about an hour before the debate. JFK was alert, forceful, and energetic during the debate, and public opinion seemed to declare him the victor. After his election in 1960 and until the time of his death in 1963, he continued to periodically use Dr. Jacobson's cocktail either by injection or by sublingual (under-the-tongue) drops. JFK considered Dr. Jacobson's cocktail necessary for his well-being.

During his Presidential campaign he, his doctors, and family attempted to secretly keep the nature of his health problems from the public. In particular, there were claims that he had Addison's Disease with the implication that it was due to tuberculosis. The effort to claim deleterious health issues didn't apparently affect the campaign, and he was elected, at age 43, President of the USA.

JFK's assassination at age 46 on November 22, 1963, brought about a medical controversy that in the minds of some is still not settled. The issue is whether he was killed by one or two bullets and whether they were shot from his front or back. The four treating physicians at the Dallas Parkland Hospital, who tried to save him, and the two pathologists at the Bethesda Naval Hospital, who did his autopsy, all agree that two shots from the rear dealt the death blow.

JFK's medical records were made available to a few of the nation's top historians and medical investigators beginning in 2002. His records and new scientific medical knowledge have combined to determine that the underlying cause of JFK's basic, lifelong health problems was principally a rare disease called "autoimmune polyglandular syndrome." JFK's autopsy revealed that both of his adrenal glands were almost totally absent. This evidence confirmed that autoimmunity destroyed his adrenal glands and gave him Addison's Disease. To complicate matters, he appeared to develop a rare spinal condition called "adhesive arachnoiditis" caused by a toxic myelogram dye which was injected into his spinal canal. JFK's popular and idolized political career that ended in a tragic assassination has diverted attention away from his health issues. A close analysis, however, reveals that he had a strange, one-of-a-kind medical saga.

20. Medical Chronology

MEDICAL CHRONOLOGY		
DATE	**AGE**	**EVENT**
May 29, 1917	0	Born with a shortened leg, unstable back, and autoimmune polyendocrine syndrome.
1917 – 19	1-2	Starts incessant childhood infections. Severe case of scarlet fever.
1920 – 30	3-13	Bronchitis, chicken pox, ear infections, German measles, measles, mumps, whooping cough. Bruises easily. Gastrointestinal symptoms.
1931-36	14-19	Appendectomy. Weight loss, failure to grow, joint pains. Diagnosed with colitis or duodenitis – today called celiac disease. White blood cell count lowers to dangerous level. Leukemia suspected.
1936	19	Football injury starts lifetime of back pain
1937-38	20-21	Started on liver extract and possibly deoxycorticosterone for gastrointestinal symptoms.
1938 - 40	21-23	Pain starts in sacroiliac joint and back after playing tennis and football while attending Harvard University.
1943	26	PT109 incident. Back pain flares.
June 23, 1944	27	Major spine surgery at Lahey Clinic, Boston. Little or no pain relief. Doctors mystified.

1945	28	Declared permanently disabled and discharged from the Navy.
1946	29	Elected to Congress.
1947	30	Diagnosed with Addison's disease by Sir Dave Daniels in London. Given last rites on return to USA.
1947 - 50	30-33	Deoxycorticosterone (DOCA) and cortisone started by Dr. Ephraim Shorr, endocrinologist.
1950-51	33-34	Collapsed with severe infection in Okinawa, Japan.
Sept. 12, 1953	36	Marries Jacqueline Bouvier.
1952 - 55	35-38	Elected to Senate. Back pain progressively worsens, and legs weakened. Crutches required.
Oct. 21, 1954	37	Second back surgery. Double disc fusion, bone graft, metal plate inserted. No help with pain or weakness. Given last rites.
Feb. 10, 1955	37	Surgery to remove metal plate and wound debridement.
May 26, 1955	38	Dr. Janet Travell starts a comprehensive pain and rehabilitation program. Diagnosed with pernicious anemia, and hypothyroidism.
1957	40	Pain and weakness reduced to a point that JFK can start to campaign for presidency.
1957	40	Dr. Gene Cohen becomes his endocrinologist.
Sept. 1958	41	Developed wound abscess and required

		incision and drainage.
1960	43	Family and campaign deny presence of Addison's disease. Seeks out Dr. Max Jacobson for stress and weakness. Takes Dr. Jacobson's cocktail before Nixon debate.
Jan. 1961	44	Dr. Travell appointed White House Physician. Drs. George Burkley and Gene Cohen are also White House physicians. Dr. Max Jacobson continues care.
May 1961	44	In Ottawa for tree planting ceremony. Bends over and back goes into severe, disabling spasm.
Oct. 1961	44	Dr. Hans Kraus brought to White House for physical therapy.
June 1963	46	Resumes playing golf.
Oct. 1963	46	Tells Dr. Kraus he will go without corset in 1964.
Nov. 22, 1963	46	Assassinated. Overall health best in his adult life.
1992	0	Adrenal atrophy confirmed. American Medical Association reports that two bullets shot from above and rear killed JFK.
2008	0	Dr. Lee Mandell determines that genetic "autoimmune polyendocrine syndrome" is basic cause of JFK's major medical conditions.
2019	0	Dr. Charles Burton determines JFK had adhesive arachnoiditis due to a

		myelogram dye. Provides a reason for severe back pain and failed surgeries.

21. Selected Bibliography

1. Addison T. On the constitutional and local effects of disease of the supra-renal capsules. *Samuel Highley*, London, 1855.
2. Aldrete JA. Arachnoiditis: the silent epidemic. *Future Med*, Birmingham, AL, 2003.
3. Altman LK, Purdum TS. In JFK file, hidden illness, pain and pills. *The New York Times*, Nov. 17, 2002.
4. Blair, J. The search for JFK. *Berkley Putnam*, New York, 1976.
5. Bumgarner JR. The health of the Presidents. *McFarland & Co.,* North Carolina, 2004.
6. Crenshaw CA. JFK conspiracy of silence. *Penguin Books*, New Your, 1992.
7. Dalek R. An unfinished life: John F. Kennedy 1917-1963. *Back Bay Books*, Little, Brown, and Co., 2013.
8. Dalek R. The medical ordeals of JFK. *The Atlantic*, Dec. 2002.
9. Ghigo E, LanFranco, Strasburger CJ. Hormone use and abuse by athletes. *Springer Science*, New York, 2011.
10. Graden PJ, Livingstone HE. High treason: the assassination of President John F. Kennedy-what really happened. *Conservatory Press*, Brooklyn, PA, 1989.
11. Hersh S. The dark side of Camelot. *Bay Back Books*, New York, 1997.
12. Kerr R. The practical use of anabolic steroids with athletes. *Robert Kerr*, San Gabriel, CA, 1982.
13. Lertzman RA, Birnes WJ. Dr. Feelgood. *Skyhorse Publishing*, New York, 2013.
14. Lifton DS. Best evidence: disguise and deception in the assassination of John F. Kennedy. *MacMillan Pub Co.,* New York, 1980.
15. Livingston HE. High Treason II. *Carroll and Graf Publishers, Inc.* New York, 1992.

16. McMahon EB, Curry L. Medical cover-ups in the White House. *Farragut Publishing Co.*, Washington, DC, 1987.
17. O'Brien M. John F. Kennedy: a biography. *Thomas Dunne Books*, New York, 2005.
18. O'Reilly B, Dugan M. Killing Kennedy. *Henry Holt & Co.*, New York, 2012.
19. Pitts D. Jack and Lem: John F. Kennedy and Lem Billings: the untold story of an extraordinary friendship. New York: *da Capo Press*, 2007.
20. Reeves TC. A question of character: a life of John F. Kennedy. New York: *Macmillan*;1991:92-3.
21. Schwartz JEB. JFK's secret doctor: the remarkable life of medical pioneer and legendary rock climber Hans Kraus. *Sky Horse Publishing*, New York, 2012.
22. Schwartz S. Into the unknown: the remarkable life of Hans Kraus. New York; *iUniverse*;2005;177.
23. Sorensen T. Kennedy: the classic biography. *Harper and Row*, New York, 1965.
24. Tennant F. Clinical diagnosis and treatment of adhesive arachnoiditis. *Tennant Foundation*, West Covina, CA 2022.
25. Travell JG. Office hours: day and night – the autobiography of Janet Travell. *World Publishing Co.*, New York 1968.
26. Travell JG, Simons DG. Myofascial pain and dysfunction: the trigger point manual. *Williams and Williams*, Baltimore, MD, 1984.

22. Medical References

1. Addison T. Anemic disease of the suprarenal capsules. *London Medi Gaz*, 1849;12:535-46.
2. Barton SH, Murray JA. Celiac disease and autoimmunity in the gut and elsewhere. *Gastroenterol Clin North Am.* 2008;37(2):411-428.
3. Bishop PMF. The history of the discovery of Addison's disease. *Prac Royal Soc Med*, 1949;43:35-42.
4. Breo DL. JFK's death: the plain truth from the MDs who did the autopsy. *JAMA.* 1992;267:2794-2803.
5. Burns CM. The history of cortisone discovery and development. *Rheum Dis Clin North Am* 2016;42:1-14.
6. Burton C. Adhesive arachnoiditis: the day they poisoned JFK. *The Burton Report* 2019;19:1-4.
7. Campbell PN, Doniach D, Hudson RV, Roitt IM. Auto-antibodies in Hashimoto's disease (lymphadenoid goiter). *Lancet.* 1956;271(6947):820-821.
8. Carpenter CCJ, Solomon N, Silverberg SG, et al. Schmidt's syndrome (thyroid and adrenal insufficiency): a review of the literature and a report of fifteen new cases including ten instances of coexistent diabetes mellitus. *Medicine (Baltimore)*. 1964;43:153-180.
9. *Dorland's Illustrated Medical Dictionary*. 23rd ed. Philadelphia, PA;WB Saunders;1962.
10. *Dorland's Illustrated Medical Dictionary*. 26th ed. Philadelphia, PA;WB Saunders;1981.
11. Falorni A, Laureti S, Santeusanio F. Autoantibodies in autoimmune polyendocrine syndrome type II. *Endocrinol Metab Clin North Am.* 2002;31(2):369-389.
12. Hartman FA, Thorn GW, Lockie LM, et al. Treatment of Addison's disease with an extract of supra-renal cortex (cortin). *J Amer Med Assn*, 1932;98:788-793.

13. Henry DE, Chiodo AE, Yan W. Central nervous system reorganization in a variety of chronic pain states: a review. *Phy Med Rehab*. 2011;3:1116-1125.
14. Krueger C. Methadone for pain management. *Pract Pain Manage*. 2012;12(2):69-75.
15. Lovell RG. Autoimmune reactions. *Current Therapy*. In: Conn HF, ed. Philadelphia, PA:WB Saunders;1965:425.
16. Lundberg GD. Closing the case in JAMA on the John F. Kennedy autopsy. *JAMA*. 1992;268:1736-1738.
17. Maclaren NK, Riley WJ. Thyroid, gastric, and adrenal autoimmunities and insulin-dependent diabetes. *Diabetes Care*. 1985;8(suppl 1):34-38.
18. Majeroni BA, Patel P. Autoimmune polyglandular syndrome, type II. *Am Fam Physician*. 2007;75:667-670.
19. Mandel LR. Endocrine and autoimmune aspects of the health history of John F. Kennedy. *Ann Intern Med*. 2009;151:350-354.
20. McEwan BS, Biron CA, Brunson KW, et al. The role of adrenocorticoids as modulators of immune function in health and disease: neural endocrine and immune interactions. *Brain Res Rev*. 1997;23:79-133.
21. Neufeld M, Maclaren NK, Blizzard RM. Autoimmune polyglandular syndromes. *Pediatr Ann*. 1980;9:154-162.
22. Nicholas JA, Burstein CL, Umberger CJ, et al. Management of adrenocortical insufficiency during surgery. *AMA Arch Surg*. 1955;71:737-42.
23. O'Leary C, Walsh CH, Wieneke P, et al. Coeliac disease and autoimmune Addison's disease: a clinical pitfall. *QJM*. 2002;95(2):79-82.
24. Pain. *The Merck Manual* 9th ed. Rahway, NJ: Merck Co. Inc. 1956;1146-1147.
25. Pait TG, Dowdy JT. John F. Kennedy's back: chronic pain, failed surgeries, and the story of its effects on his life and death. *J Neurosurg* Spine 2017;27:247-255.

26. Robles DF, Fain PR, Gottlieb PA, Eisenbarth GS. The genetics of autoimmune polyendocrine syndrome type II. *Endocrinol Metab Clin North Am.* 2002;31:353-368.
27. Roitt I, Donaich D, Campbell PN, et al. Autoantibodies in Hashimoto's disease (lymphadenoid goiter). *Lancet* 1956;2:820-21.
28. Roundtree LG, Greens. The treatment of patients with Addison's disease with the "cortical hormone" of Swingle and Pfiffner. *Science* 1930;72:482-483.
29. Schmidt MD. Eine biglandulare erkankurg (Newbennieren und Schilddrusse) bei Morbus Addison's. *Verh Dtsch Ges Pathol Ges.* 1926;21:212-221.
30. Shatz DA, Winter WE. Autoimmune polyglandular syndrome, II: clinical syndrome and treatment. *Endocrinol Metab Clin North Am.* 2002;31:339-352.
31. Swan RC, Land MB. The therapeutic value of the rocking chair. *Lancet* 1960;276:1441.
32. *Taber's Cyclopedic Medical Dictionary.* 16th ed. Philadelphia,PA:FA Davis Co.:1989:143.
33. Tennant F. Simultaneous use of stimulants and opioids. *Pract Pain Manage.* 2011;11:10-12.
34. Therapeutic indications. *Physician's Desk Reference* 9th ed. Rutherford, NJ: Medical Economic, Inc., 1955.
35. Totsch SK, Sorgek RE. Immune system involvement in specific pain conditions. *Molecul Pain* 2017;13:1-17.
36. Travell W, Travell J. Technique for reduction and ambulatory treatment of sacroiliac displacement. *Arch Phys Ther.* 1942;23:222-232.
37. Travell J, Travell W. Therapy of low back pain by manipulation and of referred pain in the lower extremity by procaine infiltration. *Arch Phys Med Rehabil.* 1946;27:537-547.
38. Urist MR, Hudak RT, Huo YK, et al. Osteoporosis: a bone morphogenetic protein autoimmune disorder. *Prog Clin Biol Res.* 1985;187:77-96.
39. Wass JAH, White KG, Elliott A. Osteoporosis, osteopenia, and osteoarthritis in autoimmune hypo-adrenalism. *Endocrine Abstracts.* 2006;11:207.

INDEX

About The Author

Forest Tennant has spent most of his medical career as a practicing physician and researcher in the fields of addiction and pain medicine. He has published over 300 scientific articles and books in these fields. For his efforts he was given a "50 Year Achievement" award by "Pain Week." In this 50-year span he has been a US Army Medical Officer, UCLA Professor, Public Health Physician, and Drug Advisor for the Los Angeles Dodgers, NASCAR, and National Football League. He was the Editor of Practical Pain Management for 12 years. He recently discontinued clinical practice to dedicate time on the study of intractable pain and spinal cord disorders. He and his wife, Miriam, have been married 56 years and they split their residence between West Covina, California and Wichita, Kansas where they headquarter their real estate finance company, Tennant Homes. Their charitable giving and medical studies are sponsored by The Tennant Foundation. Prior to this writing, the medical history of JFK, he has written similar books on Howard Hughes and Elvis Presley.

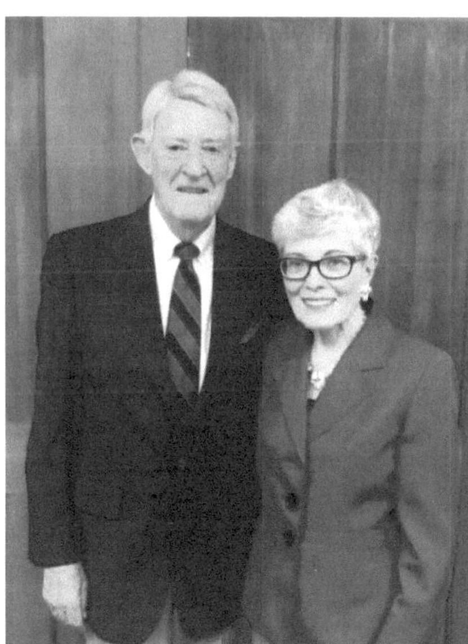

OTHER BOOKS BY FOREST TENNANT

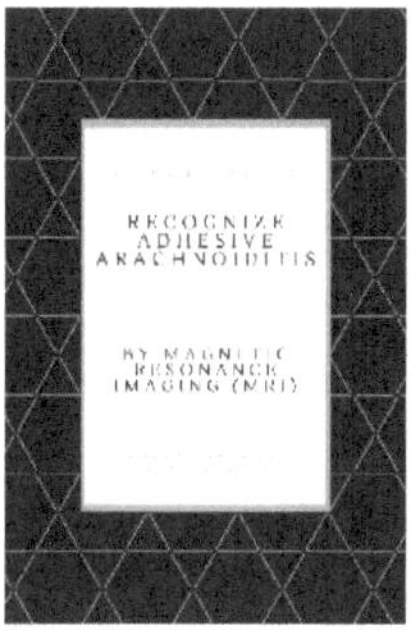

HANDBOOK TO RECOGNIZE ADHESIVE ARACHNOIDITIS BY MAGNETIC RESONANCE IMAGING (MRI)

ISBN: 9781955934152
LOC: 2021925161

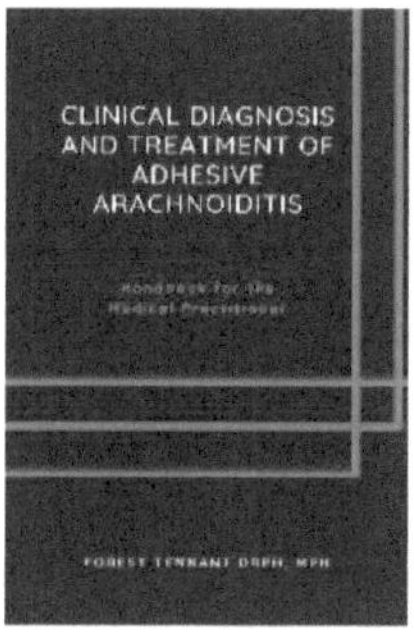

CLINICAL DIAGNOSIS AND TREATMENT OF ADHESIVE ARACHNOIDITIS

ISBN: 9781955934183
LOC: 2022907190

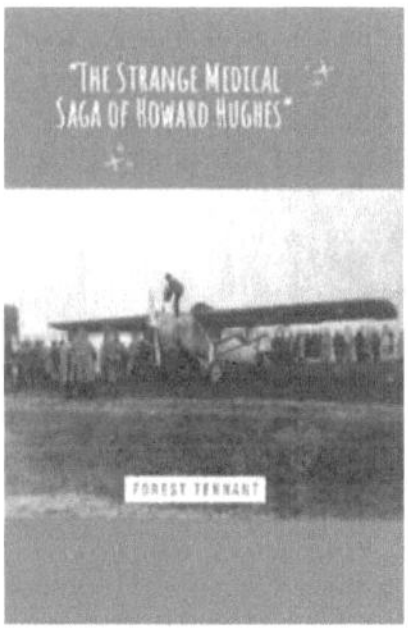

"THE STRANGE MEDICAL SAGA OF HOWARD HUGHES"

ISBN: 9781955934091
LOC: 2021912855

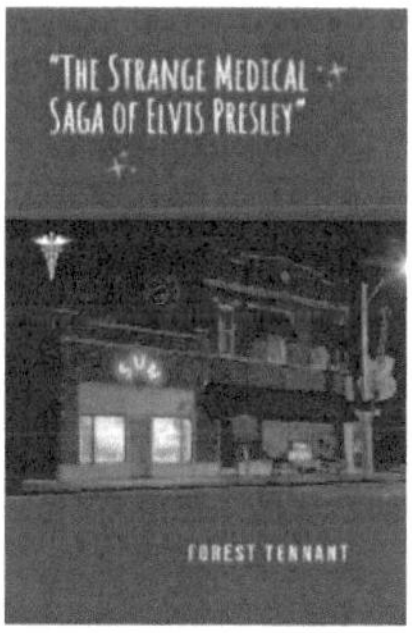

"THE STRANGE MEDICAL SAGA OF ELVIS PRESLEY"

ISBN: 9781955934008
LOC: 2021911718

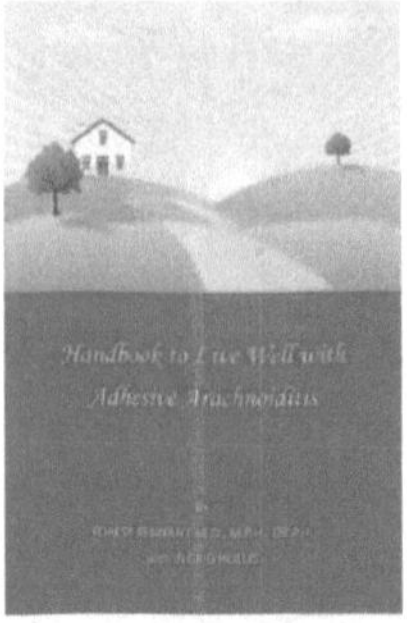

"HANDBOOK TO LIVE WELL WITH ADHESIVE ARACHNOIDITIS"

ISBN: 978195934060
LOC: 2021912718

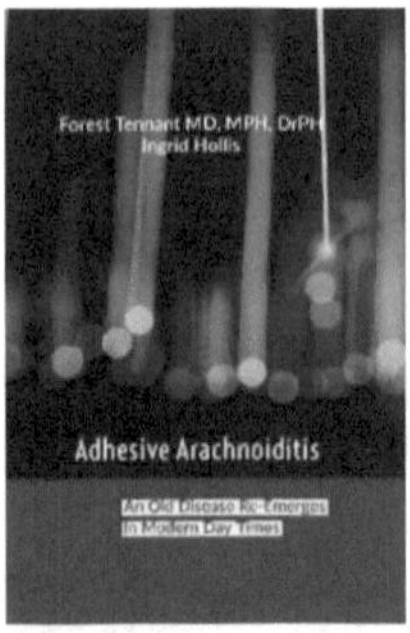

"ADHESIVE ARACHNOIDITIS: AN OLD DISEASE RE-EMERGES IN MODERN TIMES"

ISBN: 9781955934039
LOC:2021912467

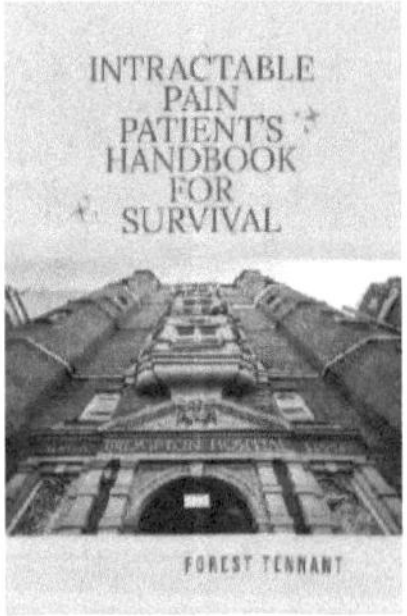

INTRACTABLE PAIN PATIENTS' HANDBOOK FOR SURVIVAL

ISBN: 9781955934121
LOC: 2021916464

Made in United States
Troutdale, OR
11/03/2026

56844876R00096